ME AND MY BIPOLAR...
FOREVER TOGETHER

ME AND MY BIPOLAR... FOREVER TOGETHER

Brigid Sheehan

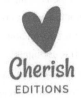

Cherish
EDITIONS

First published in Great Britain 2021 by Cherish Editions
Cherish Editions is a trading style of Shaw Callaghan Ltd &
Shaw Callaghan 23 USA, INC.
The Foundation Centre
Navigation House, 48 Millgate, Newark
Nottinghamshire NG24 4TS UK
www.triggerhub.org

British Library Cataloguing in Publication Data
A CIP catalogue record for this book is available upon request
from the British Library
ISBN: 978-913615-50-5
This book is also available in the following eBook formats:
ePUB: 978-1-913615-51-2

Cover design by More Visual
Typeset by Lapiz Digital Services

To psychologist Dr Ruth Sigal of the Women's Resources Centre, University of British Columbia, Canada, who threw me a lifeline and helped me more than she could possibly know.

CONTENTS

1   A Family of Prima Donnas   1
2   Moving House Takes a Heavy Toll   13
3   Nuns and Habits   23
4   Discovering my Genes   27
5   Blissful University Life   39
6   Living the Life in Ladbroke Grove   51
7   Two Psychiatric Hospitals   61
8   Back to Blighty   65
9   Putting Down Roots   75
10 Becoming a Parent   87
11 Giving up on Psychiatrists   97
12 Heart Surgery   103
13 Another House Move   107
14 Another Challenge: Menopause   111
15 Retirement   117

    Acknowledgements   121

ABOUT THE AUTHOR

Brigid Sheehan is a British-Canadian woman who recently retired from a decades-long career in social work with a sense of both fulfillment and exhaustion in equal measure. She lives in a leafy, semi-rural part of southern England with her partner and their two sons in their twenties. Brigid hopes that her story will resonate with you, whether you or someone you love has faced a mental health condition.

1
A FAMILY OF PRIMA DONNAS

This is a memoir about quite an ordinary life – mine – that has had
to accommodate an extraordinary medical condition, one which has
taken me to some unexpected places along the way. I have inevitably
picked up some medical theories about bipolar disorder, such as it is,
but I can only speak for myself as a patient and share insights that
are unique to me. My five siblings will have their own memories, as
seen through the filter of their age and place in the family, factors
that bring further character-building aspects. Formal diagnoses of
bipolar tend not to be made before the late teens, but I wonder if
the die was cast for me much earlier. Did childhood traumas, big
and small, dent my resilience, or did genetics alone play a major
role? Perhaps it was a combination? Does the key to understanding
it lie best with psychiatry or psychology? Maybe a more integrated
approach would have helped me.

It's probably best to start at the beginning, or thereabouts. The
summer of 1963 was a watershed time in my seven-year-old life. As
I sat on the concrete steps at the back of our new house in South
Croydon, I gazed across the valley towards London, thinking that I
could see Hillingdon, where everything I had ever known had been
left behind. I must have been told about the move, but not necessarily,
or perhaps I chose not to pay attention. As the fifth of six children
in the family, things did not always get explained, and it was often
assumed that everyone knew everything. I had a pain in my chest
whenever I sat on those steps, which was often. I would think about
my two best friends, never to be seen again. For a time I would talk

to an imaginary friend who lived inside the steps and was amazingly called Nehemiah Bultitude. One day my mother tried to talk to me about her after hearing me call her name. It broke the spell and seemed to help me move on, but I was deeply wounded for the first time in my life by the seismic change of that summer.

Life originally began for me in 1955 with a home birth at 46 Corwell Lane, Hillingdon. My eldest sister Frances is ten years older and was born in Queen Charlotte's Hospital at the end of the Second World War. Labour took four days and, on arrival, she was blue with a bruised, pointed head. My mother recalled becoming aware that Frances was being put quietly to one side, and she insisted on having someone attend to her. She was baptized in case she didn't survive. Frances was fine in the end, but home birth was unsurprisingly the chosen option for all five subsequent babies.

My birth was unremarkable. I had blue eyes, red curly hair, and I was destined to be called carrot top in the outside world. My middle sister Clare also has red hair, but it is straight. Frances, Anthony, Brendan and John have brown hair and blue eyes. We don't particularly look alike, but we seem to share some facial expressions. My mother always described us as a family of prima donnas because we had distinct personalities and would argue to the death about any subject at all. Our suburban semi didn't seem crowded to me, but it must have been, although when not at school, we were always out of the house in the park or further afield. There was a rope that hung from a tree down at the nearby canal that we would swing on over a bomb crater to try and hit the overhead cables. It was thrilling. I don't think anything like this would have been mentioned to our parents, although they were anything but helicopter types – a very modern phenomenon. Famously, Clare fell in the canal one day, and Frances calmly found a branch on the towpath and pulled her out with it.

Life was quite regimented, probably out of necessity – money must have been tight but was never talked about. My father worked as a clerk for Nestle, and my mother was a teacher who had to give up her career when she married. Bath night was on Friday and taken in turns. Washing day was Monday, when all the beds were changed, and my mother manned the twin tub with grim determination. Changing beds was hard work in the days before duvets, but I liked the feeling of being tightly tucked in with blankets. By the end of the day, weather permitting, shirts were ironed and on the airer, while the airing cupboard was filled with sheets and towels. I still love the sight of a full washing line billowing in the wind. I don't think people changed their clothes as often as they do now, and it certainly would not have been feasible for a household of eight with limited resources. We each had one pair of Clarks shoes and a pair of wellingtons that were in continuous use during the long, snowy winter of 1963.

All meals were eaten at the table. We had cereal for breakfast every day except Friday, when we had baked beans on toast. Lunch on Saturday was shepherd's pie, and something was roasted on Sundays. There was always a pudding: spotted dick, jam roly-poly or a suet jam pudding called Boiled Baby, which was cooked in sheeting material. Everything was homemade, with date fingers, scones, coconut haystacks, gingerbread or diggers for tea with bread and butter. We drank lots of milk and water. At least once a week we had stew, which was my favourite. On the day my younger brother John was born – a tremendous shock to the system for me at age four which, again, I don't think anyone told me about – my mother rose up from her bed, got out the pressure cooker and made a stew. She reached up for the salt on the overhead shelf but got hold of the Vim instead, and she shook it liberally into the pot. Taking a moment to consider this, she just stirred in the cleaning powder, and nobody seemed worse for wear. Mum was 46 when John was born and probably extremely tired. She mentioned once that when Anthony was born, a home help appeared courtesy of the new welfare state, but by the time she had six children, there was no help. Later in life she explained that she constantly made the same meals because there were so many likes and dislikes that she just stuck to what she knew eight of us would eat.

On Saturdays we always went to change our books at the library. Without a television, reading was really great. I could escape into a book and shut out the general hullabaloo. I loved Enid Blyton. We did get an old TV from my Auntie Celie in around 1962, but using it required everyone taking turns to hold up the aerial and follow instructions from the rest of us on how to maintain a grainy black and white picture. We would watch black-and-white war footage of *All Our Yesterdays*, and *Doctor Who* became an exciting favourite. Like hundreds of small children all over the country, John would hide behind the sofa as soon as the music started.

Trips to the library were accompanied by trips to the sweet shop, as Saturday was also pocket money day. We each received a penny per year of our ages. This bought a surprising amount of sweets: pineapple chunks, rhubarb and custards, dolly mixtures, and liquorice comfits measured out from glass jars, weighed and put into paper bags. From the sweet shop we usually went home via the swings in the park, which we regarded as our own. I loved dangling from my legs on high bars above the concrete and making the roundabout go wildly fast.

We had one notable exception to our Saturday routine when my father took us to watch the Campaign for Nuclear Disarmament – also known as the "Ban the Bomb" march – that proceeded along the Uxbridge Road on one side of the park. It left quite an impression on me. Mum and Dad both felt that one shouldn't disclose how one voted or how much one earned, but there were sometimes clues to their individual political leanings. When President Kennedy was assassinated, Mum gathered us in the living room to say a Hail Mary, probably more because he was a Catholic than a Democrat.

Our Saturday outings did not generally include Mum, who may have been trying for a bit of peace and quiet, but both Mum and Dad would lead the whole family on what came to be known as the Sunday route marches. We would walk for miles. Dad would carry homemade lemonade in glass bottles, which predated plastic and were heavy. He would dispense carefully measured "daddy drinks," just big enough to make you long to have your thirst quenched. Coming across a fountain was a wondrous experience that seldom happened. We didn't have a car, so walking had no novelty value. In fact, our garage was rented out to a man called Mr Moody until Clare and I found his black Ford car unlocked and we played at driving. Whatever we did, the car shot into reverse when he next turned on the engine, and the rental arrangement was terminated shortly thereafter.

Sunday mornings always involved mass at the local Catholic church. We wore our Sunday best, which, for me, included hats and coats with velvet collars. We had some very nice clothes, which our cousins passed down to us. But dresses were homemade on my mother's manual Singer sewing machine, and my sisters and I learnt dressmaking from her using paper patterns from McCall's. My mum also made clothes for our toys, which were played with a lot and valued. We scrubbed up well with shiny shoes and took up an entire pew in the church.

The mass was still celebrated in Latin, and this seemed to give it a power and mystical resonance that didn't really carry over when it was later translated clumsily into English. Other changes were on the way. At first, the nuns who taught us wore full square wimples around their chins and floor-length black habits, which gave the impression that they glided silently like machines. Seeing them a few years later in knee-length habits and veils that showed their hair and faces was not only a revelation, but also a much more practical, comfortable and less scary fashion choice. The church had a beautiful painting, *Immaculate Heart of Mary* by Pietro Annigoni, above the altar. When the long masses seemed unending and the sermon proved impenetrable, I would often find myself mesmerized by the serpent in the painting being crushed under Mary's foot. All of my siblings except for the youngest, John, attended Botwell House, the primary school attached to the church. Some of the buildings were cold, temporary post-war blocks. For lunch we walked in a line across the road to the civic restaurant, another wartime resource, where we ate alongside mostly male manual workers. It is the only place that I ever recall routinely serving half a fried egg to children.

I later discovered that one of the priests was quite an entrepreneur, making some extra money for the church by holding rock concerts. One day as Clare and I studied a poster of the Rolling Stones pasted outside the school, we decided they were very ugly in comparison to The Beatles. It was a frequent debate in the early 60s.

I don't think there was much play in the school curriculum, and we seemed to work quite hard at copying letters and numbers. I took to it straight away. There was physical punishment, and I can remember the sensation of a ruler on the palm of my hand or the flicker of a soft slipper. Why this would happen to me, I cannot imagine, although I was very chatty at that time. My mum said that I would talk to her all day long in my preschool days and that she was going to miss me when I started school. She listened to *The BBC Light Programme* on the wireless a lot, and I always disliked it when I heard the theme tune from The Archers, as I knew from her faraway look that she would be lost to me until it finished.

Years later, Mum told me that when she was washing the kitchen floor, she could see planes going over, as we were quite near Heathrow Airport. Spotting them would make her think that she would never be a passenger on one. There was a lot of drudgery for a mother of six at that time. Feminism didn't yet hang in the air, although the battle of the sexes was certainly being enacted in our house, with constant cries of "Not fair!" In the run up to any major events, particularly Christmas, Mum would hum, rub her hands together and loudly say things like "Rimsky Korsakov" or "Madre De Dios." We were used to it, and it seemed to indicate that well-contained stress was boiling over. Right up until she died, Mum had a card by the kitchen sink that said, "Our Lord, Thou knowest how busy I must be this day. If I forget thee, do not thou forget me." It was written by Royalist General Jacob Astley as his battle prayer at the battle of Edgehill in the First English Civil War.

John was a small toddler who was constantly falling over and bumping into things, resulting in a perpetually grazed nose on his very handsome face. He once spectacularly pulled the bicycles outside the kitchen door down on himself, and there were five or six as everyone rode one. I should have played more with John, as he sometimes seemed like a separate family of his own, but I was always drawn to the others who were older and, therefore, more interesting. John did not speak until he was three, but my mum was unconcerned. When he did start to talk it was in whole sentences. We probably all interpreted for him and he didn't feel the need to speak. When I started school, Mum would push John in his pram and bring our dog Penny on her lead down to the main road where I would get the bus. The trio would meet me from the bus at the end of the day during that first year. Sometimes, I would be with my siblings, but I think they must have had different timings in the juniors.

One particular occasion arose when I walked home alone from school after a grim incident. At the end of the day, the class stood in a circle to say a Hail Mary. I had put my hand up and asked twice to be able to go to the toilet, but Mother Mary Oliver told me to wait. Halfway through the prayer I could wait no longer, and a stream of wee crashed onto the wooden floor and spread noisily. I was taken to the medical room and given a pair of boys' grey flannel trousers to wear while my knickers were rinsed out and wrapped in newspaper. I don't think a word was spoken. I decided that I couldn't get on the bus because everyone would see the boys' trousers hanging below my tunic. I rushed home as quickly as I could on foot and came through the door in a complete fury, throwing the newspaper on the floor and trying to explain what had happened. When my mother picked up the newspaper, it was empty, which meant a pair of thick navy knickers was presumably somewhere on Botwell Lane. It wasn't really anger that boiled up but shame... a horrible emotion.

On the whole, I loved school and my two friends, Jane and Susan. I made my First Confession after being taught that there were three basic sins to confess and, thereafter, I just left out anything that didn't fit. Holy Communion followed, and I basked in a very simple sense of right and wrong. Hell, devils and ghosts were a major deterrent to sinning, and Heaven was the goal – simple. The school year was punctuated by Christmas, Easter, Bonfire Night and a holiday on the South Coast. An annual summer holiday always took place during the last two weeks in August, and we would take a train to the coast in an operation planned with military precision. My mother would rent a house from *The Lady* magazine, and we took all the sheets and towels in my dad's army scatter bags. We spent a couple of summers on the Isle of Wight, sharing a house with my Little Auntie Lucy and two of my cousins, Mary and Tim. There was a croquet lawn, and we would unintentionally knock seven bells out of each other's knees with the mallets. Sitting on the beach with sandy sandwiches and looking in rock pools was bliss for me, although, as most of my siblings were growing up fast, interest was probably starting to wane. One unwelcome aspect of beach holidays was sunburn from which Clare and I suffered badly, despite being told to wear t-shirts. Calamine lotion was used to calm down the heat and stinging that plagued us at night, and on one occasion my mum put a fireguard in my bed to keep the weight of the blankets off me. Red skin and red hair was not a good look. We would peel off each other's burnt skin. We had no idea of the risks.

At the end of the summer holidays, Christmas started to come into view. The Christmas tree went up on Christmas Eve and came down on the Epiphany, by which time Mum had had enough of it. My dad managed to put presents from Father Christmas on the end of each bed without anyone ever waking and seeing him. We had stockings with an apple and a tangerine, plus other gifts. We each bought seven presents to give, and that took some budgeting from our pocket money. My dad would say he just wanted good behaviour for Christmas and would end up with six plastic combs. The crib was put out in its straw, and a candle burned all night in the window to light Our Lady on her way. The Christmas cake and puddings containing sixpenny pieces and silver charms wrapped in foil were made in November. School nativity plays monopolized hours of school time along with carol singing. My mum took a lot of trouble with the Christmas tree and would hang sugar mice that would soon lose their ears. I always enjoyed mass on Christmas mornings, as it was uplifting, but really we just wanted to get home and start the festivities.

Easter always seemed a more serious religious festival, and Good Fridays were dour, but our main concern was eating chocolate eggs after Lent. Bonfire Nights were great fun with a bonfire in the back garden and lethal Catherine wheel fireworks that could go in any direction. My mum would make hotdogs and cups of Milo, a malt drink that Dad would get from the Nestle staff shop, along with bags of misshapen chocolates. It always seemed slightly strange to me that Catholics would celebrate a failed gunpowder plot and the execution of the Catholics involved. It was frowned on by some people at church, but we had a great time. As there were eight of us, we were always a crowd and tended not to have outsiders involved. I used to feel very awkward and shy around visitors to the family home.

Generally, we played lots of games at home, from dressing up and board games to hide-and-seek and murder in the dark. Clare had a doll called Marigold and a toy panda. I had a doll called Rosebud and a teddy called Edward. We would spend hours playing in our bedroom with the twosomes and imagining all sorts of scenarios using the special high-pitched voices we had for them. Brendan and Anthony made a go-kart from old pram wheels, and they had a big dug-out in the back garden that was covered with my dad's army cape. No one was allowed in – they armed themselves with catapults – so I have no idea what they did there.

We had a gang of friends at the park who we roamed about with after school. I also had a tiny friend called Sandra who lived a few houses down. She had a tin of biscuits and bottles of fizzy cream soda under her bed, which seemed extraordinary. It was my first experience of a fizzy drink – out of this world. Sandra's mother always smelt of the Guinness that she drank ostensibly for health reasons, and her father was a small, angry bullet of a man whose dinner had to be on the table within 20 seconds of him coming in the house. With hindsight, I'd say there were a few issues there. One day he suddenly took Sandra and I in his van to a circus. We were squashed in the front passenger seat before the dawn of seat belts, and he drove fast. I thought the poor, miserable animals seemed sad, and the clowns were awful. Mum was very worried, and I was forbidden to go to Sandra's again, which seemed a bit unfair, as I had never wanted to go to the circus in the first place. Clare and I used to visit a set of elderly neighbours after church each week, and they would slice a Mars bar in half for us. This arrangement ended abruptly when Clare asked if she could have a whole one. That was the extent of my social circle. Sometimes our paternal grandmother quietly came to stay, and, mostly at Easter, Big Auntie Lucy was a very unwelcome addition to the household. Strict and opinionated, she would rule the roost, and we had to have salad every day. A tall Victorian woman, she would wear large black hats with hat pins, and she would comb out her long, silver hair on the landing at night while singing hymns in a reedy voice.

In the year before we moved house, Mum took me to see my paternal grandmother in Islington, where she lived alone in part of a large rundown Georgian house. All the buildings in London were black with soot at that time, and it made them look ancient. My grandmother was called Bridget, and she wanted to see me because we shared our name, although my spelling was different. I have spent a lifetime dealing with people insisting on correcting the spelling for me, but Brigid is one of several Irish spellings.

My grandmother was in her late 70s when I went to visit her in Islington, and she had made a tiny jug of red jelly for me to eat. I was captivated by this. Bridget was Irish and came from a prosperous family who had lived in a hamlet near Castlebar in County Mayo. She was destined for a life of looking after two wealthy maiden aunts but sought adventure instead, running away to London where she became a domestic servant. It must have been a brave and perilous journey. Clare visited Killadeer near Castlebar a few years ago and found the shell of the family shop still standing. She spoke to friends of distant relatives in the pub who knew the tale, and she said she felt she was having a genetic memory, as she looked like everyone there. Clare does strongly resemble photographs of our paternal grandmother.

Bridget met and married my grandfather Patrick, a master plasterer who drank so much that it had a dire impact on the family's fortunes. There are some sepia studio photographs showing him looking very intense in a sharp Edwardian-style suit, bowtie and dark-rimmed glasses, surrounded by Bridget and the children, who all seem stiff and constrained. Patrick was a choirmaster, but he must have had a random musical gene that was not passed on to anyone else. Dad would recall being sent to get his father out of foul pubs, but he was not critical of him.

My dad was the eldest of five children, and he was born in Belgravia in a house that still stands and is beautiful now, but it probably didn't look that way in 1914. The family went to Dublin for the next ten years because my grandfather said he would not fight for the British Army. With IRA connections, he had some involvement in the Easter Rising of 1916. On their return to England, the family lived in slum dwellings in London and had a tough time. Dad and his brothers would spend hours playing football out in the streets. He could remember very little about his childhood in Ireland, only the porthole on the boat as they returned to the UK. Later in life Clare gave him a recording of *Angela's Ashes,* and he could barely bring himself to listen, so I expect the themes of poverty and deprivation had resonated with him.

Dad struggled at school and always thought of himself as unintelligent, although it was evident that this was far from the case. He left school at 13 and delivered pencils in the City for Eversharp. Dad would have liked to have had a trade, but his father was set against this, so he attended The Working Men's College to learn shorthand and typing. It had a sports ground and gave him opportunities to play team sports. He and some other students also got to travel to Germany at a time when their culture was highly regarded, although Hitler was already on the rise. Dad saw him from a riverbank as he travelled to a rally by boat.

Dad's qualifications were to prove useful during the Second World War. The Army had a shortage of troops with clerical skills, so Dad spent most of the war in the West Country as a motorbike dispatch rider and then as a corporal. He took good care of the men in his platoon and would help them write letters, as many could not read or write. On Friday nights he played cards with them and always won, but would take the winnings to buy everyone fish and chips. In many ways it was probably a good experience for my dad after the life he had lived previously, although D-Day and its aftermath proved a challenge. Namely, he got separated from his unit, so there was a long delay in sending the telegram to my mum to let her know he was safe.

My grandfather died in middle age. The maiden aunts left a spiteful will that excluded my grandmother. Their money went to Bridget's brother, who had spent most of his life in California working as a butler and never married. He accumulated some money himself and helped Bridget out at times. He died shortly before Bridget and left everything to her but, sadly, she died before seeing any of it. My dad's share helped us to buy our next house. Bridget went into hospital quite soon after we saw her, and Dad would visit her. One day he had a bottle of orange squash to take, a rare sight in our house, but after he had left the hospital called to say she had passed away. Without mobile phones we couldn't contact him, and I couldn't bear the sadness of him arriving at the hospital to find she had gone. When he got home all I could think to say was, "Where is the orange squash?" Children so often say the wrong thing at times of heightened emotion, and Dad just said gently that he had given it to the nurses. Bridget was buried in Kensal Green Cemetery on an exceptionally cold day. Dad took Anthony and Brendan, who recall wearing short trousers in the bitter wind at the graveside.

2
MOVING HOUSE TAKES A HEAVY TOLL

My childhood in Hillingdon in the 1950s and early 1960s was
not absolutely perfect, but it seemed very happy indeed. I never
really warmed to 15 Heathhurst Road although, in time, it came
to be a splendid house lovingly decorated by my dad, who was
very proud of it. We had moved to South Croydon because Nestle
relocated there and paid for us to do the same, and the timing of
the inheritance from my paternal grandmother enabled us to have
a bigger house. The exact location was chosen because there were
good Catholic schools plus a Catholic GP and a Catholic dentist.

Our new home was a roomy four-bed Edwardian semi with tulips
on its stained glass windows. Inside, it had a strong smell of cats
that hung around for months, and the decor was just strange. The
living room had a different wallpaper pattern on each wall. Plus, the
house had been divided into flats and roughly converted back. The
dining room was interesting, as it had a trap door in the floorboards
with wooden stairs leading down to the cellar. The brick walls were
whitewashed, and there was enough headroom for my brother
Brendan to have it as his den. Next door was a coal cellar with a
chute located at the top of the kitchen steps, where the coal deliveries
on the back of the coal man would be counted in by the bag.

The breakfast room was the hub of the house where we gathered
to eat and get warm around the boiler. For a time we also had Little
Auntie Lucy's parrot Malachi in a large cage in the breakfast room.
He would spit seeds and screech in quite a bad-tempered way. One
day, we found his cage empty with the back door open. Nobody has
ever shed light on how this happened, and he was never seen again.

As the house was built on a hill, it had great views from the back, and the front looked up toward our neighbours across the road who were quite snobbish and territorial members of the residents' association. An alleyway ran through the houses to the railway station, and commuters would often park in our road and walk down. Our neighbours not only put notes on their cars, but glued them onto the windscreen. It led to some lively exchanges, which may be why I have always disliked notes. There was little warmth from the neighbours, as far as I could tell. They may not have been keen on a large family moving in. The woman next door was acidly condescending and would put an occasional mound of rhubarb on our doorstep, as though dispensing alms. One day Clare and I were having an admittedly unacceptably loud argument in the back garden that resulted in someone slipping a letter of complaint through the door. My mother was cross with us for behaving badly but incensed that this was an anonymous letter. She said there could be no greater evil, and she bravely took it round to a number of neighbours to discuss it. I don't know what she would have made of social media.

In the road below ours, a large family of Plymouth Brethren followers had recently moved in and told my mother that someone had put contraceptives through their letterbox, which they found upsetting. It was generally a quiet road in the leafy suburbs, but one night I woke to a lot of screaming, and I could see that a man was hitting a woman in a car outside. All of the curtains opposite were twitching. I woke Brendan, and he went down, but the car moved off as he came into sight. Our neighbours surfaced soon afterwards, and I was disgusted to hear them saying that they were the residents and should not have to put up with such noise. No concern for the woman who was being battered and my expectations just got lower. Domestic violence was very gradually making its way onto the national agenda, but it had yet to reach Heathhurst Road.

Starting school at Regina Coeli meant I had to wear a new green-and-brown uniform and catch a minibus to school from the end of the road. On my first day I nervously surveyed the old house with a sweeping wooden staircase and bars on the upstairs windows. I was in a class of 46, and the room was set out in rows of wooden desks with sloping lids and seats attached. There was barely room to move, so we didn't. The teacher had complete command at the front, and that felt strangely secure. I was given a desk at the back alongside two pretty Asian girls, who became my kindred spirits, and a boy who smelt of carrots. I think I was quite shell-shocked and remained deeply homesick for my old school.

Each afternoon there was some form of activity, such as country dancing and even dancing the maypole, which broke up the day pleasantly and provided respite from the desk situation. The playground was a very busy place with long skipping ropes that could take ten or so jumping in. Football, hopscotch, jacks and various chasing games were played. There was also a curious practice of bringing in scraps with things like pictures of cherubs to swap and keep flattened in a book. I kept quietly out of the way and tried to merge with the wall during that first year.

As summer approached, things slowly began to get better. We were outside more, and Sports Day gave me a chance to show that I could run fast and win, raising my profile and giving me a bit of confidence. We did not have homework or after school clubs, so there was less pressure and space for a more free-range existence in the parks and green spaces close by. Then things really changed for the better when I made friends with Julie, who is still a good friend after more than 50 years. Julie lived in our road, and I had seen her with her two sisters walking past in red coats, their ponytails swinging behind them. They also had a baby brother. The family had lived in Singapore for several years before coming back to England, and, at first, Julie had been placed in the school year above her chronological age. However, she was moved back down and put into my class, and Julie and I became inseparable.

The minibus seemed to disappear over the summer, which was probably for the best because it was old and the back doors kept flying open. The three-mile walk to school was great. Along with siblings we gathered up various friends along the way and would chat about anything and everything. Julie's house at number 45 became my second home and quite a refuge from all the teenage angst at number 15. Julie's parents had warm Lancashire accents and they seemed very glamorous. They smoked, had a car and looked to me like John and Jackie Kennedy. At my house I think the family could be described as one of high emotion. Arguments over the bathroom, a missing piece of clothing or who had eaten the icing off someone's cake would escalate into hideous rows and acts of revenge. I took every opportunity to get away.

Julie and I got matching red roller skates that we loved. Although an unsophisticated design and probably highly dangerous, we would skate like the wind up and down Heathhurst Road for hours. We would go on trips to the little parade of local shops that included Mrs Dunbar's Bakery and Smokey Joe's, the sweetshop where it was hard to see or breathe. Joe always wore a smart cream canvas jacket and stood up straight among the confectionery, but his face was yellow, and he could hardly stop coughing as smoke curled up over his shoulder from the cigarette always hidden behind his back.

Before transferring to his office in Croydon, my dad continued to work in the City and would often comment on how lovely the fresh air was when he got off the train at Sanderstead. He probably never stopped by Smokey Joe's. The only Black person in the neighbourhood was the station manager Wally, who was quite strict with children but a witty man who liked a joke. Some people complained about him playing calypso carols at Christmas, which seemed mean-spirited.

We had lots of unpleasant childhood diseases, and I seemed to get them all: two types of measles, chickenpox, scarlet fever and whooping cough. I recall staying in Frances's bedroom at these times, away from everyone else in a sort of quarantine. I liked having my mum come in and stroke my forehead. Although there was emotional warmth, there was very little physical affection shown in the family, so this was precious. I think my parents had quite a Victorian upbringing themselves, and some things were just not talked about. When my period started I had no idea what was happening. My mum said that she would talk to me about it, but she never did. It fell to Clare to get me organized and deliver some lurid explanations.

There was an unfortunate event that took place soon after we moved to the new house. A young man was cleaning the upstairs windows, and he asked if I wanted him to lift me up to look out through the tulip windows. I did, and he sexually assaulted me, although all I knew at the time was a pleasant, unfamiliar sensation. I stopped him from lifting John up. I told Clare what happened and said she was not to tell Mum, which thankfully she did. Mum said nothing, but I felt better knowing that she knew, and I am sure we never had a window cleaner in the house again. The significance of this event did not fully dawn on me until some years later when I understood more about sex and realized I had been sexualized. I felt dirty and guilty. It left its mark. I understand my mum's modus operandi of "least said, soonest mended", but there were times when it was definitely unhelpful.

It felt like my siblings were going separate ways following the house move. Clare started secondary school at Saint Anne's College, a convent grammar school right at the end of our road, where I was doomed to join her a few years later. Brendan had spent a year at Gunnersbury Park School in West London, where he was punished endlessly. He had to do lines for yawning in class, which was probably the result of staying up late writing lines the night before. My mother sometimes did them for him. Transferring to Saint John Fisher Grammar School, where his rugby skills gave him kudos, alleviated his misery, and he was much happier. Frances stayed at her convent grammar school in Hounslow, Gumley House, because she had only a year to complete in the sixth form, so the travelling seemed worth it, but it meant she was not around much. Anthony's situation was slightly different because he did not pass the Eleven-plus exam. In Hillingdon he went to a very rough secondary modern called Springfield Road, where most of the teachers were former probation officers. After the move he went to St Thomas Moore, a local Catholic secondary modern. My mother said she had never realized Anthony was struggling until it was too late. It was not obvious from his speech and keen mental reasoning, and he would say that he was just not interested in school.

On the whole we benefited from the grammar school system. Scholarships gave us the social mobility and access to higher education that we could not have afforded. Still, a crude dividing line damaged the self-esteem of those who failed the Eleven-plus, and it left no way forward for late developers. There were school friends who I never saw again when they went on to secondary modern schools, and it seemed very divisive.

John did well as an all-rounder at Regina Coeli and won the school cup before going to St Joseph's College in Upper Norwood. During his time there it became a comprehensive school, which meant they didn't take in pupils based on their academic achievement levels. The differences between all of us seemed greater in the teenage years, and it made me miss the cohesiveness of Hillingdon. Somewhere it dawned on me that I didn't embrace change and that change was inevitable.

In my junior years at Regina Coeli, Julie's friendship was a constant that was very important. Clare and I had always had an intense relationship from which we both needed to move on. We confided in each other about everything, and I trusted her implicitly. We shared a small double bed until Clare went to college, so there was literally no space between us. Clare was clever, angry, creative and very amusing. I would try to defend her at times or negotiate our way out of crises that seemed to blow up on a daily basis. I simultaneously wanted to be there with her and to get away. It was probably the same for her.

Regina Coeli became an oasis that was warm and friendly. The work seemed to require little effort, and I had a sense of attainment. The nuns were kind and approachable, although there were occasions when they made some odd choices. One day the whole class had to walk across to the nearby Catholic church with no explanation and found a coffin, something that many of us had never seen before. It was a requiem mass for the father of a boy in our class and his sister. There were whispers that he drank. As we were the only mourners, I think it was a really nice idea for us to fill the church, but a bit of preparation and a note to our parents would have helped. At that time nuns and priests tended to think that their authority trumped that of parents, and the emotional needs of their pupils did not register at all. The two children whose father died disappeared for good, and I wonder if they were taken into care or, hopefully, moved to other family members.

There were children from lots of different backgrounds at the school, and all we had in common was being Roman Catholic. Quite a lot were Irish or of Irish descent and would spend summers in places like Kinsale, which sounded brilliant. We did not have any Irish relatives that we knew of. Wearing a home-knitted cardigan or a non-uniform coat could mark you out for a hard time from the nuns, who were often terrible snobs. When I went on to grammar school, I missed the vibrant variety of characters and found everyone, including myself, middle class and rather boring. I was developing an inverted snobbery.

Frances went to teacher training college in London and would appear at home from time to time looking slim and sophisticated in miniskirts. It was the swinging 60s. I remember her trying to introduce me to a yogurt that tasted horrible. I didn't discover rice or pasta until I went to university. I missed Frances, and her departure changed the dynamic at home, as she had always held a certain reassuring authority as the eldest. I visited her in London sometimes and remember seeing a demonstration against the Vietnam War in Hyde Park. Frances was head of her student union and often went on marches. She was also brave enough to bring boyfriends on her visits home. We would sit around the dining room table and watch them closely. The man who Frances would later marry managed Sunday lunch with us, then ran with her to the nearest pub for a stiff drink.

Anthony left school at 15 with a Certificate of Secondary Education in Religious Education and began an apprenticeship at a local garage. Before that, he had excelled in wood and mental work. He also held the distinction of having knocked out the actor Bill Nighy in a school boxing match. Very on trend, he wore a parker and rode a scooter. My mother replaced the fur on his parker with a much bigger piece. Anthony liked to go to dance halls with his friends, and he would emerge from the bathroom in a cloud of Old Spice in preparation. Brendan played a lot of rugby with the school team and made a firm group of friends. He went on to Plymouth Polytechnic to study geography and reappeared during holiday times as a changed man with a beard, a Bob Dylan hat and a West Country accent. I think he was actually styling himself on the folk singer Ralph McTell. Clare, John and I remained in full-time education for the time being.

Julie and I became fashion-conscious with our short skirts and identical, treasured red Dr Scholl shoes. *Top of the Pops* and *The Man from U.N.C.L.E.* made Thursday nights mandatory for the telly. The first time Jimi Hendrix appeared singing "Purple Haze", the playground was buzzing the next day. We had never seen anything like him. Our other great love was The Monkees. A school friend whose family were really quite hard up splashed out on buying Julie their LP for her birthday. When asked if she had a record player, Julie was quite overwhelmed and said no, but she just wanted to hold the record. On Friday evenings Julie's dad would take my dad in his beloved Borgward car – complete with plastic still on the red leather seats – to Cater Brothers food shop in Croydon's Surrey Street Market for a weekly shop. Julie and I often went along to pick up substandard fruit and veg from the ground while the market stalls were being put away. When we got home, we would get out the scales and set up our own market, charging our parents outrageous prices.

John had a good time at school and was becoming a footballer. As he was four years younger than me, I didn't see a lot of him, but I can claim to have saved his life there once. John wandered up to me one day and told me that he and his friends had eaten peas from a tree. I told a teacher, who alerted the parish priest, Father Rodell. He was one of the few people with a car, so he took John and his friends to Mayday Hospital for a stomach pump. As it turned out, the peas were Laburnum seeds, which can be lethal to children if they eat 15 or more of them.

When Julie suffered her first migraine, the school secretary seemed not to understand and told her to go to the medical room. Instead, Julie decided that, if she was going to die, she wanted to be with her mother, so she snuck out and walked home. The go-to man, Father Rodell, was duly dispatched to find her in his Morris Minor, where he probably spent much of his time on emergency duties, but she made it home before him. In juniors year three Julie and I joined Girl Guides and went on camping trips that were an experience – mostly of damp musty tents, latrines and feeling cold. It was fun to be with a group of girls nonetheless. We also had guinea pigs for a short time at number 15 and number 45, but they were cruelly killed by foxes. Clare and I were looking after Julie's guinea pigs while they were on holiday, and we felt very responsible that they also died. When they got back we bought them a little white albino replacement. Soon afterwards, that one was killed, too, and Julie's dad couldn't bear any more grief. Although the guinea pig was cold and quite stiff, he put everyone in the car and took it to the People's Dispensary for Sick Animals so the vet could pronounce it dead. Another burial followed. Events like these punctuated my childhood and taught me so much.

I was really sad when our days at Regina Coeli were drawing to a close, as I knew the pain that was coming in terms of endings. We did have a brilliant class outing to Littlehampton that summer after the Eleven-plus. I'm not sure how Julie and I managed to walk on the pebbles with our long white socks and Scholl sandals, but we made it onto the beach for a picnic. Strict instructions were given not to go on the Big Dipper in the theme park, but, within seconds, a naughty boy called David was seen up on the ride shouting about how slow it was. Suddenly it dipped very fast and we could see the whites of his eyes. Nobody else ventured up there. The sun was shining, and we had a great time.

3
NUNS AND HABITS

Another change of school involved another change of uniform, one that was particularly grim this time: a smoky blue pleated skirt and matching blazer with a coffee-coloured shirt, topped off with a blue felt hat that looked like an army helmet. It wasn't designed for redheads – or anyone, actually. The school outfitters were Hewitts in Crown Hill, Croydon, where they seemed to think I would be growing a lot, but it never happened, and my uniform remained roomy. Clare had already been at my new school, St Anne's, for four years, so I knew a fair amount about it, and none of it was positive. I felt sick on the first day and disliked the smell and darkness of the corridors. The food, prepared in the basement by two enormous nuns, was truly horrible. I wasn't keen on it being an all-girls school and missed the warm informality of Regina Coeli. There was a two-form intake, and Julie and I were in separate classes, which immediately cast me adrift, although there were other familiar faces. On day one, I saw Clare and her friends telling some of the new first years to kneel at the founder's portrait, and I quickly dissociated myself from this mischief. Following in an older sibling's footsteps can be problematic in terms of expectations. Later in the year, Clare got her hands on a bunch of keys and rang the Angelus bell to sound an emergency alarm, and she and her friends locked several classrooms, including mine, causing a minor panic. I just knew it was Clare, but she wasn't caught.

The impact of changing schools had quite an immediate effect on my self-esteem and my capacity to learn, as I found it hard to concentrate. At the end of each month, there were monthly tests in all subjects, and each student's average mark determined the colour certificate they received and their place number in the class. I slid through gold to pink to green rapidly and very publicly, as our teachers called us to the front to receive our certificates in order of merit. Used to doing well in all subjects, I was bewildered. Maths and Latin lessons seemed to go on with no engagement from me at all. It was like a long slow nightmare, particularly as Latin was taught by the headteacher, a nun who terrified me. I sat at the back of the class and started to make friends with a little group of three girls who seemed quite different and basically marginalized. They all travelled on the bus from South Norwood and had gotten to know each other en route. Unlike their classmates they were not comfortably middle class, but they were bright and interesting. I maintained my friendship with Julie, and we played netball together, but I was moving in a different direction. At the back of the class with my new friends, we would make sarcastic jokes and limit our participation. We developed a dark sense of humour that we referred to as our manic-depressive sense of humour without really knowing what that meant. Winding up the nun who taught religious education with impossible questions was probably quite mean. As one tedious lesson drew to a close, she noticed that someone had put a cheese sandwich in the hand of the wall-mounted statue of Our Lady. The bread even had a large bite mark corresponding with Mary's mouth and a smaller one for baby Jesus. I have no idea who did it, and nobody else had noticed it, but we all had our bags searched for bread and cheese crumbs.

These sorts of things would happen, and they often left me feeling as though I was in a strange, other-worldly institution, which, of course, I was. Keeping a grip on reality was difficult as time went on. In my early teenage years, I tended to feel numb and anxious. My hands would shake, and I dreaded having to answer a question in class because my voice would just disappear. My thoughts would turn in on me, and I am surprised that I was able to learn anything. I disguised it as best I could by seeming aloof and remote out of choice. Added to this I felt very ugly with my frizzy red hair and freckles. Sometimes Clare would help me with homework, but this was not always a help. She was good at art and offered to finish my drawing of John Wesley, but replaced his Bible with a frothing pint of beer. I didn't notice and, fortunately, neither did the teacher, who gave it a tick. My only redeeming skill was playing netball well, which meant I could wear a team sash with my uniform. It seemed like a protective factor in a sea of girls who could be quite unpleasant if they sensed vulnerability. I also found security in my small group of friends, who could hold their own in an environment that they equally disliked. We started to spend time together after school and on weekends. We would take the bus to Croydon and meet up with some older boys from another Catholic grammar school in a coffee bar. We soon became cigarette smokers. I loved smoking and have missed it since the day I gave it up. It probably had a calming effect. Attitudes were very different then. Going to the GP involved sitting in a waiting room with everyone crowded round a giant ashtray in a blue fuge.

A watershed in terms of developing our style came when we bluffed our way in to see the film *Easy Rider*, an 18, and we left the cinema as hippies. All things American seemed great at the time. We also became fans of The Faces and went to a great concert at The Greyhound in Croydon. They were our band until "Maggie May" was a hit, and then they belonged to everyone. The world seemed to be opening up. Pubs in South Norwood became our stomping ground, and I would just tell my mum I was staying with my friend. As the fifth child my siblings had paved the way for me to have more freedom. I also was not great company at home around this time, so was probably not greatly missed, in truth. Saturday jobs provided money for cigarettes and drinks. We often drank a bottle of Mateus Rose or Blue Nun while getting ready for the pub. It gave me a sort of confidence, although I would invariably slide into the background at the bar, nursing a drink and hoping nobody would notice me. After last orders we would all go back to somebody's house and listen to music. Neil Young, Lou Reed and Bob Dylan's *Blood on the Tracks* were favourites, and joints would be passed around while we listened. I didn't smoke marijuana, as I didn't like feeling out of control, although I didn't experience the same sensation with alcohol. We would stay up all night and go straight to school in the morning, feeling absolutely grim. I finally had more of a teenage identity, but I remained desperately shy and often felt miserable for no apparent reason. Young men were interested in me, but I would freeze them out as though they didn't exist. Basically, I had no idea how to speak to them. I felt out of sync with the world, and I don't know how apparent this was to other people, but I must have seemed a bit of an oddball. Every teenager probably recognizes times like this, but I have a feeling this was magnified for me. When I was 14 Clare left school and went on to the same teacher training college that Frances attended. I was desperately sad that she was going – I felt she was my security – but once she had gone, it felt as though a weight had been lifted. I had lots of conflicting feelings and a powerful sense of loss. The course and career choice of teaching did not suit Clare. She dropped out, to use a popular expression at that time, and moved to Scotland, then to Cornwall with a friend, before returning to London a couple of years later. My favourite coat disappeared with her but did come back eventually.

4
DISCOVERING MY GENES

My mid-teens were a more positive time. Saturday jobs gave a bit of
independence and structured the week, and I generally enjoyed the
work. My first job was at a large department store, Allders, in Croydon,
where I was put in the soft upholstery department – not something
I had a wide knowledge of. The first customer had a diagram of her
furniture that I could not fathom. She was elderly and kept shaking
her stick while addressing me like a domestic servant. Dissatisfied, she
moved off, and my experienced colleague emerged from tidying under
the counter to say that she often came in and needed to be avoided.
I learnt that some customers want to bolster their sense of superiority
at your expense, and colleagues don't always have your back. At the
end of a very slow day, I received a meager pay packet (take out with
10 shillings inside as this was pre-decimalization), which barely covered
my bus fare. I arrived home in despair and told Anthony that I had
signed a contract with Allders. He said that no contract is binding if
you are under 16, and I felt so relieved. One of the good things about a
large family is that there is always someone around to help.

My next Saturday job was at a bakery called Willsons. They
sold fabulous bread, cakes and pastries that would arrive by van on
wooden trays to be put on the shelves while still warm. It was a busy
shop with lots of hilarious banter between staff and customers. Pre-
decimalization meant I needed to use some nimble mental arithmetic
before ringing up the clunky till. After the lunch rush hour, the part-
timers would go home, and I would be left on my own for an hour,
during which time an elderly man would always come and look in

the window for ten minutes before coming in and asking for two rock cakes. He looked like a private person and quite down at heel. I would put in a few cream cakes that were unlikely to sell at that time in the day. He would never mention it, and neither would I. When Clare left school she bequeathed me her Saturday job at a hardware store in Croydon called Turtles, as it paid much better than the bakery. I always seemed to follow in her footsteps. It was an extraordinary shop that sold absolutely everything and is much missed. Staffed with interesting characters, I enjoyed the working environment. During my time there decimalization came in, as did the introduction of Value Added Tax (VAT) at 10 per cent. Jeremy Turtle decided that the VAT could easily be added on at the till but didn't reckon with the fury of shoppers who reasonably expected to pay what was on the price tag. People were throwing down so many purchases that we eventually had to come in on Sundays to stocktake and re-price everything.

Holiday jobs provided money to travel. I worked at IBM two summers in a row, at first as a call despatcher, taking details from customers about their computers and passing them onto engineers. Computers in the 1970s were quite large and unfamiliar to most people. My colleagues would take useful messages like "modem down," while I would record that the computer had sort of blown up and there was smoke, or something of that sort. It became a bit of a comic turn not to be repeated. The next year I worked in IBM's restaurant wearing a green dress overall with a tiny white apron and frilled cap. One of the older executive men would come down at quiet times to try and persuade me to go away with him. I had to dodge around the tables to keep him at bay. These were the days when women were regarded as fair game, and I must admit I almost expected such passes because of popular culture at the time. TV shows like *On the Buses* and *The Benny Hill Show* set the tone at a very low bar so low that they were dangerous in undermining women's safety. Feminism was often minimized and ridiculed, although its voice was getting louder. I sought out different reference points by reading books such as *If They Come In The Morning*, edited by Black Panther Angela Davis, and following the now-controversial career of Erin Pizzey, who founded the first refuge Chiswick Women's Aid. The play *Cathy Come Home*, which aired on the BBC in 1966, opened everyone's eyes about homelessness, including mine at just 11 years old. There were other publications, such as *Up the Junction*, that helped women start to have a sense of solidarity.

I spent a gruellingly idle month working at the gloomy Department of Health and Social Security DHSS office building in Elephant and Castle. I did the job of a civil servant named Rodney that took 30 minutes a day. I recall Conservative politician Ken Clarke describing it as a terrible building, and I found it positively debilitating with its labyrinth of tiny corridors and box rooms. Lunchtime trips to the lively East Street Market on Walworth Road provided some relief. Once that ordeal was over, I went on a 12-hour coach trip with my three friends to Dundee, where we rented a cottage from someone's aunt for a fortnight. In the middle of nowhere, it was very boring, but we just liked the independence.

This time in my life felt better and outward-looking. I had learnt how to style my hair with a hairdryer, and putting mascara on my golden eyelashes made a big difference. I had to give up netball in order to have a Saturday job, but that felt fine. At school I was becoming much more interested in the work, maths aside, as we started to prepare for O Levels. Politics and arts subjects began to have more relevance to life. One Scottish history teacher brought a socialist perspective to lessons. I am sure the nuns would not have been happy, had they known. We talked about apartheid in South Africa and Northern Ireland, which were the big concerns of the day, alongside poverty, class and sex discrimination. Because we went to Catholic schools, it was years before I realized that most English people had very different attitudes towards Northern Ireland. While not condoning violence, there was an alternative understanding of the Catholic and Protestant history through the centuries that led up to The Troubles. At home we had always had lively discussions at the table with a wide variety of views. Clare loved a debate and would invite Jehovah's Witnesses into our house, despite strict instructions not to do so. My Uncle John, Mum's brother, and Auntie Maureen,

Dad's sister, came to stay from South Africa, as they were considering moving back to the UK to retire and wanted to test the waters. They had met at my parents' wedding and gone on to marry, emigrating soon afterwards. Both talked about black people being happy in their homesteads when we raised the question of apartheid, and there was no meeting of minds. After they left my mum said that, although she did not agree with their life in South Africa, she didn't think they would be able to adjust to life back in the UK.

With last-minute cramming I passed most of my O Levels, managing reasonable grades. My friends did, too, so we went on to the sixth form together. There was an unsympathetic cull of all those who didn't do so well, and they received no vocational guidance, either. The year began for us with a trip to the Careers Library, which only contained university prospectuses. One of my friends had decided to follow her brother, who was doing law at the London School of Economics. He looked like Jimi Hendrix and proved to be quite an influence on us politically. We asked our Scottish teacher if we could do the politics A Level, which was a first at the school, and she agreed. We also requested to do art history with an interesting teacher who took us to galleries and inspired us.

The sixth form was set up with small groups of tables in an informal style instead of desks, but I still remained out on a limb with my friends. During a general election in 1972, we put up Labour and Socialist Workers Party posters that were pulled down by a near-hysterical girl who said her family would have to become tax exiles if Labour won. The other tables were solidly blue and Conservative. Ted Heath was duly elected, followed by the Winter of Discontent. Homework by candlelight was not too bad, but getting caught outside in the dark with no lighting was quite alarming. I think we all spent a lot of time in bed.

My friends and I were elected to the Saint Anne's Social Services Committee (SASSU), which seemed an enlightened organization that nobody else wanted to be in. Enthusiastically, we set about planning a sponsored walk but failed to inform the headteacher until we announced it at a SASSU assembly. We kicked off with The Who

singing "My Generation" very loudly on a record player, and the
teachers nearly fell off the bench on which they stood. We were still
able to have the walk, though. One teacher who was always very strict
and sarcastic surprisingly came to our aid by solving safety issues and
patrolling the route in her car on the day – no idea how we made that
connection. Through SASSU we also visited Netherne Hospital, one
of several mental hospitals in the area. It had been handsomely built
in Victorian times with long, dark wooden corridors, where patients
looked lost in isolated armchairs. Most shocking was the powerful smell
of urine that really didn't need to be there. We were some years away
from Care in the Community 1989, which allowed for the treatment of
disabled people in their own homes, but the need was already obvious.
SASSU was a source of real education to us.

Meanwhile, our social life continued in much the same way with
pub nights and grungy, impromptu parties in South Norwood. We
had trips up to London, visiting places like Biba in South Kensington,
and Frances introduced me to the world of spectacular fashionistas
on the Kings Road. There was a brilliant viral campaign all over
the West End one summer with mysterious posters that said, "The
Godfather is coming." Eventually the book about the mafia appeared,
and everyone had their head in a copy.

In the sixth form we were able to sign in the register ourselves or
get someone else to do it, a system that did not encourage attendance.
During that year a difficult series of events arose for one very close
friend who left school – and our social circle – abruptly. It was a huge
loss, and I found myself slowly disintegrating. By this time John was
at secondary school, and my mum went back to teaching part-time
in the mornings, leaving early in Anthony's mini and picking up his
workmates on the way to Caterham. She loved having a lift, but the
smell of oil and yesterday's clothes on the other passengers nearly
knocked her sideways. With the house empty I spent very little time at
school, and I would stay in bed late. It felt like a sort of paralysis, and
I don't know where the time went.

I still wanted to go to university, and I applied to do sociology
at Lancaster. It was a really popular course in the 1970s, although

often derided as not being a real academic subject. I was invited for an interview and, although I could have spent the night in the halls, Clare arranged for me to stay with some of her friends to give me a real experience of the place. This turned out to be a freezing squat with students who had dropped out and couldn't understand why I would want to join the establishment. I barely ate or slept. Actually, there was nowhere to sleep, but somehow I got through the interview. The interviewing panel were amused by the quite derogatory comments from my school statement but said they did not take too much notice of nuns. I think it probably helped, and I was offered a conditional place.

The rest of the school year limped on after that. I had missed a lot of work, but I borrowed notes and essays to try and get ready for the exams. School just seemed to end afterwards, and I didn't go back in or say any goodbyes. Clare was living in Crouch End and her flatmate had left to get married, so she suggested I leave home and come there. The idea had immediate appeal, so I went. However many times things did not really work out with Clare, I always thought they would. It was a dark little basement flat with a shared bathroom and a leaky water heater that smelt of gas. I didn't know anyone nearby, but the idea of living in North London seemed good. I had often stayed for weekends with Clare, and we would enjoy going to places like Hampstead Heath, Kenwood, Alexandra Palace and Highgate Cemetery on the rare days when the densely overgrown old part opened to visitors. I had to get a job to pay my share of the rent and, thanks to the job centre, I went to work at a glue factory. My decision-making was just not good at the time, and I felt strange. I wasn't sleeping and had to clock in at 8am. The work exhausted me. Plus I sat next to a very needy woman who would spend all morning talking about how she loved her husband – and all afternoon about how she hated him.

Clare had started a job in the music business and was out a lot. Alone in the flat in the evenings, I found myself feeling isolated and anxious. I used a payphone to call home and get my A Level results. Brendan answered and was quite downbeat but sympathetic because he knew that my grades were not good enough for Lancaster. I felt a jolt of disappointment, and I think it was the straw that broke the camel's back. The following weekend I went home, and my parents arrived back from a rare overseas holiday, about which they had been very excited. I just burst into tears and heard my mum say something about things always going wrong when she wasn't there. I was very thin and looked terrible. She was comforting, and I went off to bed, where I seemed to stay for months, apart from seeing the GP. I remember John coming in, waving his hands around and saying Brigid's gone mental. I looked at him, and he realized immediately that it was not a joke.

The GP declared that I was suffering from exam depression, probably made worse by the glue factory job, which he clearly found incomprehensible. He prescribed me a tricyclic antidepressant called Tryptizol to take in the morning and Valium, a benzodiazepine, to take at night. I didn't like the sensations or the idea of taking drugs. I knew of another local girl from St Anne's who had committed suicide with prescription drugs intended to treat her depression. For a time my mum counted the tablets to make sure I was taking them. I seemed to be in a stupor much of the time and occasionally thought the television or radio was talking to me. My family tried to make sense of all this. I remember quite lucidly telling Mum that I might as well be in the Maze Prison, then hearing her tell someone on the phone that Brigid thought she was in the Maze Prison. One day my dad told me that we were going to the GP because I was queer. That really came out of left field, and I told him it was ridiculous and I was not going. I could only speculate that my dad thought I was having a relationship with my friend who left the school. An older, devout Catholic, Dad really would have worried about this, but I don't know what he expected from the GP.

I was allowed to smoke in my room; my mum probably thought I was suffering enough without stopping me from smoking, too. Anthony brought me a duty-free box of cigarettes, although they were Embassy rough-cut ones, so he may have had aversion therapy in mind. I smoked them anyway. Brendan let me listen to his records in the cellar, but I played *Bridge over Troubled Water* so often that it became a bit of an obsession and didn't help my grip on reality, plus I scratched the vinyl. The worst part was that I woke up each morning thinking I was better and, within half an hour, the numbness and sadness would re-emerge. Time drifted by, and I felt a sort of physical pain all of the time that I couldn't quite locate. When I am depressed I frown, and two deep lines appear between my eyes. They are still a tell-tale sign that helps me understand what is happening. But at the time, I didn't know anything about the illness. I didn't know when or if it would end or whether it would get worse. It was really helpful to have a visit from my two remaining school friends. One of them had suffered clinical depression when her father suddenly lost his sight, and she talked about how depression is a very selfish thing because you cannot think of anyone but yourself. She also pointed out that if it was a physical illness or injury, people could see and understand it, but a brain illness cannot be viewed. When I felt as though I would always be in this state, she would tell me that it was the illness talking. Just hearing that someone I knew had experienced this nightmare made a real difference, although she had to keep repeating these things over time when I didn't have any hope. It's hard to analyse a period of depression because it makes no sense but is intensely painful until it is gone, and there are no significant memories from it worth holding onto.

Months earlier my two school friends and I had arranged a holiday in a caravan somewhere near Bournemouth, and we decided to go ahead. It was a disaster for me because I couldn't cope with the change of environment, and the rain tapping on the roof all night was torture. One night my heart seemed very fast and was pounding alarmingly. I think I was probably losing track of my medication and taking too much or too little. When we moved into the caravan, we could not find any cutlery until one night I made a cup of tea in the early hours and left a teaspoon in the sink. The following morning everyone was mystified, and I could not recall where I had discovered it. We never did find a cutlery drawer, although I clearly had at some point, and it left me feeling hopeless and incapable. We went to see *The Three Musketeers* at the cinema, and the noise and massive screen overwhelmed me so much that I couldn't concentrate. On the way back to the caravan, I was stopped by a policeman who checked my details on his radio to see if I was a missing person. I must have appeared to be in a drugged-up state. My friends were great and there for me all the way through, although I don't think any of us knew what this holiday was going to entail, and they probably had a terrible time. Getting home was a relief as always, and I had to start recovering all over again.

As the months went by, I didn't really seem to be getting any better. The GP arranged for me to go to a day centre to see a psychiatrist. I think my mum was worried that I wouldn't go, so she arranged a taxi and tried to talk it up as an experience. I went and found myself in a basket-weaving situation with several doctors observing a lot of catatonic patients. They said I needed a new prescription but did not explain what it was or what it would do. The psychiatrists themselves seemed strangely detached and remote in their white coats. The whole event made me very cross and energized for the first time in a long time. I took myself to the GP to tell him that I did not want basket weaving or any more medication. He said that he had hoped this would be the result, although I think he was making that up. We agreed that I should stop the medication and start getting out more. He probably did tell me to reduce the drugs gradually, but I just stopped. I was left with shaking hands and sweating, but I was determined to get over the withdrawal symptoms.

I got myself a temporary job as a clerical assistant at the Department of Health and Social Security office in Croydon. It was the lowest rung in the civil service ladder, so I had a chair without arms. Shuffling case files around was very mundane but perfect because it did not require effort or contact with others. I learnt to avoid all eye contact, and I think I just felt too ashamed and worried that somehow people could tell I had been mentally ill. The caseworkers were seeing plenty of mentally ill claimants at the counter, so it would be quite familiar to them. However, having the structure of a job and something to get up for was what I needed and all I could cope with at the time.

I was functioning better but still very run down and lacking confidence. Regular meals, sleep and staying occupied slowly helped me back to health, and I was lucky to have my family behind me. I think it was hard for my family to know how to help. Anthony gave my mum some money to take me shopping for a new dress, and the gypsy-style one I bought from Miss Selfridge was my favourite for years. Being interested in how I looked was a good indicator of recovery. Brendan thoughtfully bought me a rug-making kit that someone had recommended, but I didn't use it, as it seemed too much like occupational therapy. When my clerical job came to an end, I spent some time back at Turtles. I felt quite self-conscious, as I had been through a life-changing experience, but the staff members there were all the same. I didn't feel able to share what had happened, and this made me wonder how I was going to manage what I came to know as the stigma.

I was nevertheless starting to think about future plans. Julie came home from Bangor University with her brown hair blond and listening to Joni Mitchell. She was having a great time, and I decided to apply to Warwick to do history and politics. My choice of subjects was partly determined by the fact that I have no maths O Level and never passed a maths exam in secondary school. The joint degree did not require maths, as statistics were not a large part of the course. Today it would have been a major barrier in both my education and employment. A lot of able people with all the right qualities get excluded from jobs as a result of rigid criteria.

Julie's friend Jackie was at Warwick, and I went to stay for a weekend to see if I liked it. I loved it. I made an application, and my mum went to see the headteacher at St Anne's. This was a big deal, as Mum had respect for her fellow teachers and for nuns, but she insisted that they write a new reference for me and said that both of her daughters had been let down by the school. I felt really supported because I know that would have been hard for her. She seemed almost triumphant when she got home.

My mum talked to me about Auntie Celie, her sister who was my godmother. I had no idea that she suffered from severe mental illness and spent periods in hospital. She was a small, pretty woman who was always nicely turned out, and she made perfect pastry. For birthdays and Christmases she would send me Bronnley soaps. I often received letters on blue note paper, mostly about her dog Biddy or my cousins and Uncle Jack. I felt really sad for her. She had a close friend who died in childbirth, triggering a nervous breakdown when she was quite young. I was used to Auntie Celie sitting with her sisters at family gatherings, chatting and laughing. She had a deep, dry voice, probably caused by medication. It seems we would only see her when she was well. I could tell that my family members had started making assumptions that history was repeating itself. It explained the remarks Little Auntie Lucy had made on a visit, clearly to check me out. Sometimes people seem to think that mental illness renders the sufferer desensitized and hard of hearing. If I had known a bit about Auntie Celie's illness, it might have helped me to recognize what was happening to me, but I also think the confidentiality wishes of the individual need to be respected. I don't like to think of her in a mental hospital feeling vulnerable or having the electric shock treatment that impacted her memory. Auntie Celie had a very lined face, and I remember Dad once saying to me that she was the youngest sister but looked the eldest because her life had been so hard. I never had a chance to talk to Auntie Celie about our mental health and, unfortunately, I was in the US when she died at 60, so I missed her funeral. Mum told me that doctors had warned early on that the drugs she had to take would impact her longevity. We probably would not have had a discussion because she was a private person, but I feel she reached out to me with all her letters.

5
BLISSFUL UNIVERSITY LIFE

By the summer of 1975, I felt recovered from the depression that had dominated much of the year. Life would never be entirely the same again, in that I'd had a profound experience that changed my perceptions. I now had something in common with other mental health sufferers. However, I had no expectation that I would face depression again, so I don't think I had a particularly good understanding of what had just happened. It was a good summer, going out with friends and having a bit of money to spend on clothes that were long and hippyish. At the pubs that we had long frequented, my friends knew about my depression. They had seen me once or twice in a bewildered druggy state when I tried unsuccessfully to manage a night out. Some people were quiet and unsure, but most really welcomed me back and acknowledged that I had been through a tough time. I think it is a little bit like bereavement: it is hard to know what to say, but it's so welcome if you just say anything.

That summer I enjoyed shopping trips with Mum and visits to the theatre and other places of interest. Going to an exhibition at the Imperial War Museum had an unexpected outcome when wartime songs started to play and Mum fled to the exit in distress. She said she did not want to think about the war and all the sad things that had happened. I knew that Mum hated the blackout that took place during some of her best years when all she wanted was to be out dancing to big bands. She had lost friends, too. Mum had trained to teach primary children, but during the war in London, she taught in a tough secondary school at the docks, and she would often be sick from anxiety in the mornings. She had to teach swimming although she could not swim herself, so she just kept counting the heads. At night she did fire watching on rooftops with a woman who became a good friend and painted her portrait while they were on duty.

My mother and her three sisters, Mollie, Lucy and Celie, along with their brothers, John, Joe, Gerard and Bernard, moved to West London at the beginning of the war. In terms of family history, my maternal grandfather James and his two younger siblings were placed by the magistrates' court into industrial schools in 1894 when they were found wandering the streets of Newcastle. Their parents were convicted of child cruelty and drunkenness. Catholic industrial schools were spartan care institutions where children learnt a trade. James trained as a gardener, and his brother was taught to look after pit ponies. James went on to obtain a position in a large household, where he met and married my maternal grandmother Elizabeth, who worked as the ladies' maid. He was punching above his weight. James ensured that his sister, who had been placed in a separate industrial school at the age of two, was installed as his new wife's replacement. Their brother was also working close by. Clearly a caring man and a survivor who knew industrial schools were harsh institutions, James took his young family to try their luck in Canada.

My mother was born in Hamilton, Ontario, in 1915, which has enabled me to have dual citizenship. After some bleak years the family decided to return to the UK. Big Auntie Lucy was keen to see them back, not least because she harboured hopes that Mollie would become a nun, a traditional path for the eldest sibling in a Catholic family. They settled back in Hartlepool, and James joined the Royal Air Force, where he trained as an engineer. The family continued to grow. Mollie, Lucy and Mum trained as teachers, and Celie as a nursery nurse because their father told them they needed a profession. My mother would have preferred to attend art college in Manchester.

The boys were mostly younger, and Bernard was only five years old when my grandmother died. Within three months my grandfather was called up by the RAF to serve in the Second World

War because of his engineering skills, and he had no choice but to go. He was stationed quite a distance away from home, and it was there that he met and married a younger woman who worked in the Navy, Army and Air Force Institutes (NAAFI). James suggested that his two youngest sons come to live with them, but my mother and her sisters turned down his offer and decided to move all of the family to London. It must have been a tumultuous time, effectively losing both parents and their home during a war. My mother never returned to Hartlepool but would mention the fierce wind and the town's infamous hanging of a monkey; plus, she could speak Geordie. She talked about teaching children with black teeth, flea bites and no shoes. They were a relatively well-off family and probably felt resented, but a main reason for leaving was the gossip that followed her father's marriage so soon after his wife's death.

My mother may have chosen to move her family to London because they had a connection to a convent in Ruislip. Auntie Mollie was keen to become a nun, but the church advised her to wait until Bernard was older before following her vocation. This seemed an enlightened decision at that time. My mum told me that, when they arrived in Ruislip, the four sisters decided to go in four different directions to look for a house to rent. When they returned at the end of the day, Auntie Celie was sitting on the pavement crying where she had been all day. I think some form of mental illness probably plagued other family members to a greater or lesser degree. Uncle Joe was a heavy drinker who always seemed to me to be acting outrageously whenever I saw him, which was usually at funerals. He had joined the Merchant Navy and acquired engineering skills before taking his family to the Middle East, where he built bridges. I am not sure how sound his civil engineering qualifications were, though, making his accomplishments all the more remarkable. He once drove his family to visit us all the way from Kuwait in a large, white American convertible that seemed to fill Heathhurst Road. I remember my Auntie Pam having a small gold bar in her handbag that she held just in case they had problems with currency at borders.

Uncle John was a health inspector, Uncle Gerard had a pub up north, and Uncle Bernard was a probation officer in London in the 1950s who went on to be director of social services in Tyne and Weir. They were all talented people. Before I went to Warwick, I had a conversation with Uncle Bernard about going into social work. I had been interested in doing this since my involvement with SASSU, but was concerned about the very harsh way that social workers were treated in the wake of the death of Maria Colwell, a child who had fallen through the cracks of several government agencies. He shared some of his experiences in probation and suggested I think about that after university.

When it was time to leave for Warwick, a Red Star Van collected my trunk, which I had inherited from Frances, and sent it by train to a house just off the campus at the university on a road called Gibbet Hill. I was a week late catching up with it, as I was unwell. Before I left Mum said for the first time that I did not have to go if I didn't want to. I confirmed that I wanted to, and nothing more was said. I could tell she was trying to acknowledge that this might be hard without wanting to discourage me or undermine my confidence. I always appreciated that Mum never tried to hold me back or treat me differently – quite the opposite, in fact. She and Clare came to Euston to see me off, and it felt great to be going out in the world.

The student house was old and comfortable with mostly shared rooms and large communal areas. There were 16 girls and, luxuriously, a cleaner. I discovered one of Auntie Celie's Bronnley lavender soaps in my sponge bag, and it was such a comfort to use it in the early weeks. The other students were very friendly, and my roommate was a lovely Welsh girl with a great sense of humour despite desperately missing her boyfriend back home. We drank endless cups of coffee and listened to Janis Joplin because we both liked her, but it didn't really lift the mood. Autumn in the Midlands was a couple of degrees cooler than the South, and the scenery around the campus was beautiful. I wore my brown duffle coat to keep warm on the hill down to the campus. This was a standard uniform with Levis and desert boots. The male students had long hair and often droopy moustaches, and many still wore army greatcoats.

When I say that I went to Warwick, people today tend to be impressed, but in the 1970s, it was still being built and, although the maths department was strong, the international reputation that has put Warwick on the map had yet to fully develop. I am sure my cohort made some sort of contribution. The student unrest of earlier years had largely petered out by 1975, and things seemed a bit boringly conventional. One housemate was from Burton-on-Trent and talked a lot about her accent and working-class roots that she found set her apart. She went off to the campus and returned a week later having found her sexual identity and came out, which was great, but she was bitterly disappointed to say that she had not been able to find any intelligent people in the whole university. I could see that it was hard to gauge expectations.

I was happy to settle into the work and routine. Lectures and tutorials were great, and I had to pinch myself that I had made it. My personal tutor in the history department was really approachable and available, plus I was lucky enough to have him for all three years. I joined the film society and learnt to project 35mm films. I was also a sometime guest at the Jewish society after making friends with people in my Jewish history course. Some weekends I saw Jackie and her friends, often for a meal. I didn't talk about my mental health, but would instead say that I had taken a gap year. Apart from feeling it would do me no favours to talk about it, I really believed it was all behind me.

When I went home for Christmas, Dad opened the door with a wide smile. I think he wanted me to feel welcome, and he had decorated my bedroom. I had been dating someone at Warwick, and he wanted me to go up to Liverpool for part of the holiday, but I decided against it. It was lovely to be looked after at home. My standard diet of boiled eggs needed some varying, and it was probably only the fruit cake that mum had put in my trunk that had kept me going. I was able to catch up with everyone, too. Life was moving on and Frances had two children by this time. I was godmother to her youngest. Anthony had a few years seeing the world as an engineering officer in the Merchant Navy before working on an oil rig in the North Sea. Brendan was an executive officer in the Home Office, Clare was working in the music business, and John was still at school. I felt grounded to be home, but I also looked forward to getting back to my own space.

During the next term I got to know other people in my house better. My roommate transferred to Cardiff University to finish her degree and get married, which definitely seemed the right plan for her. The rest of us were mostly studying arts subjects, and there were lots of late night discussions about books and politics. Eventually, we needed to plan where we were going to live next year and, along with two friends, I applied for one of the Crackley Cottages in Kenilworth. They were very sought after, but we were successful. Farmer Crackley, as we called him, seemed impressed that I lived in Surrey and said he supposed I was in the stockbroker belt. I didn't disillusion him, as it probably helped our application, but it was far from the truth. Once that was settled, we also decided to save up and spend a month interrailing through Europe in the summer. Without too much hardship we were able to save the cost of the ticket and £60 for expenses from our grants. As members of the baby boom generation, we did not have to pay tuition fees, and we received a grant that really did cover living expenses at the time – TV, phone, internet and cars not included. We were truly lucky. With everything organized we were able to lie on the grass during the long, hot summer of 1976 and study for our end of year exams. The campus resembled a holiday camp.

None of us had been outside of the UK, so travelling on the Orient Express from Paris to Athens was an extraordinary experience. In 1976 the Orient Express was not the luxury train it had been and was to be again. We stood packed in for three days and lived on bags of muesli. Our water supplies full of purifying tablets were undrinkable. As the train rumbled through what was Yugoslavia, women dressed in black who were working in the fields waved as we passed, and it seemed as though we had gone back in time. At one stage some serious German students got on and ludicrously told us not to go to Athens because it was just stones. It was sensational. We couldn't stay long, though, as we needed to make our way to the Port of Piraeus to catch a boat. Our financial planning was completely inadequate, and hotels were not possible. We caught the first boat to anywhere, which turned out to be Paros, a small island where we spent a week sleeping on the beach. The three of us rotated places each night, as we were on a slope under a shady tree, and the one nearest the water would roll down. We swam in the warm sea and read books all day. For food we walked into the tiny town for milk, cheese and large lumps of toast. We had a small calor gas stove and teabags. I'm not sure why it felt so idyllic, but it did. We knew it was time to leave when a tourist wandered past and said our tree was smelly. We had been putting our rubbish in a bag that we hung from the branches and hadn't noticed it getting noisome.

We caught a boat to Crete and hitched all over the island. Invariably, it would be a red lorry that stopped and, as we hurtled through the mountains, the lorries would only sound their horns when they saw another red lorry with no reference to safety. There were coaches everywhere, full of American tourists who seemed to be mostly elderly and in poor health. Their holidays were much more luxurious than ours, but it seemed a shame that they were doing their overseas travelling so late in life. Many could barely walk and opted out of a lot of the sightseeing that had been laid out for them. In Knossos we tried to explain to a coach party that the throne they were looking at was a replica, but the real one was just a few feet away up a hill. Without a glance they said they liked this one better, and one man said he would never manage with his back. We weren't sure if it was age or culture that set us apart, although we shared a common language.

We slept on the beaches in Crete, but it was not as restful as Paros, and our meagre diet was starting to affect us. I remember feeling tired and getting an upset stomach. The next destination was Venice, and we found it was overwhelmingly beautiful once we had woken up on the pavement outside the station. An American tourist bought us a pizza and remarked how badly equipped we were. He said to my friend Elaine, "Even your watch is broken." She had it attached to her shorts with a safety pin. When we made it to Rome, the empty Vatican at dawn was another amazing sight.

On our return to Paris, we stayed with a friend who had an apartment. I remember having a bath and, disappointingly, my seemingly tanned skin became three shades lighter. We had lots of tales to tell and seemed to have spent all summer laughing. My mother was concerned about how thin I was and said I looked like Olive Oyl from *Popeye*, but a few square meals were all I needed.

Heading back to Warwick felt as exciting as it had the first time. Our cottage was charming, but it was possibly the coldest dwelling in England. The bathroom was extended from the kitchen and, if we could find enough 20p coins for the electric meter, we could have a bath with so much steam that it was hard to breathe. We crouched around a three-bar electric fire in the living room that warmed our faces and little else. We wore fingerless gloves out of necessity and spent a lot of time down on the campus in the warm library. Books were a precious commodity, and you had to be quick to get hold of library copies. Law students were notorious for tearing out pages from reference books under the cover of a well-timed cough. It would have been great to have had the internet and access to many more sources for history and politics. We had to produce essays that would count towards our finals, but, otherwise, the second year was not particularly pressured. When we did feel stressed there was a mini market nearby that sold almost nothing, but we would buy Madeira cake and vanilla ice cream to make a comforting sandwich. One morning I came down to what I hoped was a breakfast of biscuits and instead found some change and a note from Elaine saying sorry. We were not good at catering.

Our row of cottages was on the main road towards the university, and we could either walk or wait for the bus. One day I stuck my thumb out to hitch a lift, and a bubble car stopped. I had to jump in backwards and pull a cord to close the door. It was so old and rickety, I was terrified. There was a student that my housemates called Biggles because he was in the Flying Corps, and he would drive up and down outside, pulling up as soon as I left the house to offer me a lift. I didn't welcome the attention and sometimes they would invite him in just to be annoying. He was hopelessly posh. Clare came to stay in our freezing cottage one weekend and wore her hat and gloves all the time, even in bed. Fortunately, I had arranged things to do so we were not home that much. Clare sourced a chicken from somewhere that she cooked with all the trimmings for us, and that was so welcome. The year in Crackley went by quickly. There was a really good arts centre with a theatre on campus, and we enjoyed trips to Stratford and quite a few parties. I remember walking home from the campus in the early hours and hearing a dawn chorus that was almost deafening. It felt quite magical. I remained well mentally and enjoyed life more than I ever remembered.

That summer I had no holiday plans but went back to Mum and Dad's. Frances asked if I would like to come to Wales for a week with the family but told me just beforehand that she and her husband were having difficulties in their relationship. It was a lot to take in, as I was very fond of Nigel. His brother was also joining us. They had rented a remote farmhouse that was idyllic, but Plaid Cymru had taken down all the road signs because they were in English, so finding it was challenging. Once there, we had a lovely time going on walks with the children, and Frances baked loads of bread and croissants. We played bridge in the evenings, a first for me. I felt sad and worried – as well as cross – for Frances and the children, especially because we had such a nice time. The following Christmas Frances's husband left, and my mother brought down the hat she had worn for their wedding. She tossed it in the boiler while saying, "That's that, then." It was an iconic moment that conveyed so much. I had been Frances' bridesmaid and that summer I was Brendan's.

My final year at Warwick was spent living on the campus. I had lived with my friend Elaine for the past two years, and we felt we should move there to concentrate on our finals. Our other housemate had decided not to complete her maths degree and returned to Manchester. We moved into an ugly apartment called Tocil that housed six men and six women. We knew two of the women through our courses, and they are still good friends today. I didn't really like Tocil and found the shared kitchen quite stressful. Being on campus felt claustrophobic, and I missed the walks and greenery that always helped me to wind down and still do today. A large Sainsbury's had opened just off the campus and, in no time, the place was strewn with trollies – some even hung from tree branches. Soon enough, the store had a coin-release system installed.

There was also a very justified campaign against the campus GP, with sheets hanging from windows saying "Dan Must Go." He was a disagreeable man who would not make home visits and prescribed aspirin for everything. He gave my Welsh roommate a huge bottle of it for homesickness and to help her lose weight. She stuck it on the wall with blue tack. Things came to a head when Dr Dan refused to visit a student, who turned out to have broken his leg, so someone had to push him to the surgery in a Sainsbury's trolly.

The campus was a very different landscape from the calm of Gibbet Hill and Crackley. Individually, the other students with whom we shared the flat were nice, but the men were all from the North, and their constant criticism of southerners got a bit wearing, however justified it might have been. I felt a bit like my old housemate from Burton-on-Trent, who could not find any common ground, although it had nothing to do with intelligence. I could tell that I did not feel as confident, and my sense of self-esteem had started to wane. I was losing weight, probably because I was giving the kitchen a wide berth. Nothing dramatic, but I wondered if the honeymoon following my depression had ended, and I was slipping backwards into familiar-but-unwelcome territory. It took a lot to concentrate and keep on top of my work and, although I got a reasonable degree, I felt I could have done better. In the second year my American politics tutor had suggested I apply to do a fellowship at Wellesley College·in the US, so he must have wondered why I submitted a very poor application. In fairness we had been following the American election debates between Gerald Ford and Jimmy Carter, and those discussions really wouldn't have inspired anyone.

I had started to worry about careers from the start of the third year, and I didn't relish another major change. Elaine and I stayed up at Warwick over Easter to revise, and we went to a concert by Ronnie Scott at the Arts Centre. As it was holiday time, most of the audience were from outside of the university. I found the jazz hard to follow, and the concert was clearly not going well for Ronnie Scott, who, at one point, suggested the audience just pretend they were on the Titanic. It seemed to reflect my mood well. A more enjoyable time was when Frances and her children came to stay in a Tocil room that my friends had vacated. We had a great weekend going to Warwick Castle and having a cream tea in Kenilworth, where my nephew was so fascinated by his reflection in a silver teapot that he burnt his nose.

The finals results were listed outside of the Senate House to great excitement. Mum and Dad came up on the train to Coventry Cathedral for my graduation, which was a great day, and my Tocil roommates and I took all of our parents to lunch at an Italian restaurant in Kenilworth. I dressed carefully in black and white under my gown, but did not think about how my 1970s Jesus-style espadrilles would look in the photographs. I felt really sad about leaving Warwick and the bear and ragged staff emblems everywhere. The first two years in particular had been a time when I felt happy, fulfilled and even normal without all of the self-doubt and sadness that had plagued so much of my life.

6

LIVING THE LIFE IN LADBROKE GROVE

Mum and Dad had moved in line with their retirement plans to a
lovely two-up, two-down cottage in Warlingham that faced onto
a green and almost backed onto the local Catholic church. Dad
estimated that they could just afford to stay at Heathhurst Road,
but Mum had seen the cottage on her school journeys and enlisted
the support of Little Auntie Lucy to convince him of her plan. The
house had been a bit neglected and needed some work, but, in time,
proper central heating and fitted carpets felt luxurious after chilly
Heathhurst. I had a bedroom, and John had his bed in the dining
room, penned in by my mum's Wedgewood on the Welsh dresser
and the dining table. He went off to Liverpool University soon
afterwards, and aside from end-of-term holidays, he basically never
came back south. His accent became northern.

That summer I worked on Rhodes for Clare's manager as a nanny
to three young children aged two, two and six. It was the first time I
had flown. I had my own little house with the children overlooking
the beach. It was actually quite hard work but really engrossing. The
youngest child would bang his head against an old wooden cot all
night long, and I would just pull his feet back down until he worked
his way up again. Eventually, the cot fell apart. His mother had been
told that the head banging was his way of trying to reproduce the
rhythm of the womb. It was certainly a form of self-soothing that
deprived me of my sleep, but he was a sweet child, and I tried to
encourage his speech so he would be less frustrated. His six-year-old
brother was lively, imaginative and tiny, and he had a mesmerizing

face, which made sense, considering their mother was a model. The little girl was not related to the two boys. I dreaded visits to the house from her mother because she would be inconsolable when she left, and I wanted to say that her daughter needed to be with her and not me. I had a very limited knowledge of childcare but was learning on the job and finding it fascinating. Practical tasks, such as cooking, had less appeal, but someone else handled the cleaning and laundry. Various music business characters would sneak in at night to raid our fridge and satisfy their munchies, but I mostly spent time with other nannies, who all seemed to have a Greek boyfriend working in a bar or restaurant. I returned after three months with the best tan I have ever had and a terrible hangover after goodbye tequila sunrises at every bar in Lindos. That Greek summer was very good for me. The beauty of the island and the slowed-down pace of life raised my spirits, and looking after the children was utterly absorbing. We had to have a structured routine, and I found that suited me, as I had less time to think. The sea and the star-filled night skies seemed to work their magic as they had on Paros.

Back in the UK I found that my university friends were living in different digs around London. My friend Carol got me a job at the Army and Navy Store in Victoria where she worked. Carol's aunt had worked there for decades, and she lived just around the corner. It was a job that involved filling in account ledgers and, when anyone one left the room, someone would cry out, "Whose writing is this?" Usually mine, I recall. Carol and I set about flat hunting and ended up living in the basement of a gothic monstrosity in Forest Hill with Jennie, Elaine, John and Charlie, who all went to Warwick, too. The landlord had an interesting approach to the 1974 Housing Act and thought he could get us out easily if he made the building into a bed and breakfast. Each month a load of eggs, fatty bacon, bread and margarine would be delivered and piled up with the last lot, but we stayed anyway. It was cold, damp and dark with brown carpets and magnolia woodchip wallpaper, but it was good to be together again. I remember Carol, who was basically a Londoner, saying, "I don't know where this is, but it is not London." I was not there for long before taking up a new job that I had been hoping to get.

My next stop was Dartmouth College, a rich Ivy League School in New Hampshire, where good friends of Frances' were academics. I didn't really know what the role entailed, but I was excited to get on a flight to Boston. When I arrived, I received a message asking me to get the Greyhound bus to White River Junction in Vermont, as there had been flooding and no one could pick me up at the airport. A kind man who was in the process of driving businessmen to their swanky hotels took pity on me. He drove me to the station and put me on the right bus, which must have been very annoying for his passengers. Looking down the bus aisle, I saw what looked like rows of kippers, but they were just the huge feet of the tall American passengers on board.

Phil, my new employer, picked me up and explained that I was to be a research assistant, but they were not really ready for me in terms of their workload, so he and Carol bought me some skis and dropped me off at the local slopes most days. I taught myself to ski and rarely fell over because I was wearing jeans. They were horrendous if they got wet and froze, so I stayed upright at any cost. People on the slopes were very generous and showed me how to make a stop by snow ploughing, rather than by hurtling into trees. As time went on I improved and really enjoyed it. Because I could neither type nor drive, I was not an ideal research assistant, but I did some work and whiled away the rest of the time on the slopes. Phil led focus group discussions on sugar that I had to record and read up on myself. He was also doing research for General Motors with his students, so he had the use of a small Chevette known as the lemon. Living with the family, who were really nice, isolated me, as I didn't drive and felt a bit too intimidated to make friends with the unbelievably rich and arrogant students.

I got the chance to visit New York with one of Phil's colleagues and his wife. Scott's family were Jewish and lived in Patterson, New Jersey, where we went for Passover. Their tiny apartment was bursting at the seams with relatives who all talked at the same time. I had gefilte fish, which is not something I would make a habit of eating, but it was still a brilliant evening. Afterwards, we went to see Betsy's parents, who lived in a neighbourhood called Clermont that was to become home of *The Sopranos*. It was a big house with a massive television and bowls of jelly beans, as popularized by Ronald Reagan. Betsy's parents were Christian Scientists, and her mother belonged to the Daughters of the American Revolution, an organization of women descended from those who fought for US independence. They seemed to regard me as a bit of a curiosity, and said I was just like Lillie Langtry, the British-American socialite and actress.

Betsy and Scott then took me into New York, although they worried that their orange jeep might get stolen. At this time New York was in a bad way, covered in graffiti and rubbish. We caught a yellow cab to The Dakota across from Central Park, pretending to be visiting John Lennon, and then went down to Greenwich Village to meet some friends that Scott knew from MIT who had become journalists. We had cocktails – mine was a Manhattan – in a bar called Montana Eve, where we were able to read *The New York Times* before midnight. My overloaded head was spinning by this time, though, and I was exhausted. The journalists wanted to know my impressions of Americans, and I couldn't really think of anything to say except that they seemed so big in so many ways, which didn't go down well. On Easter Sunday we went to a golf club for a really nice lunch, then headed back to Dartmouth. I'm not sure that I properly conveyed my thanks to Betsy and Scott for giving me a great experience.

By then, my time in the US was reaching an end. The onset of spring meant there had been a rapid thaw, effectively ending the skiing season. Getting back to the UK after three months was very welcome. Despite lots of initial excitement, I had felt quite lonely and disoriented during my time at Dartmouth. It was only with hindsight that I recognized the sort of depression that is not totally debilitating, but drains the colour and joy out of life for no apparent reason. Not feeling in control of these strange fluctuations in mood made me feel unnerved. Phil took me to Logan Airport, but we were late, and

I missed the flight. With Carol's American Express number, I was able to get a flight to New York to try and pick up a connection, but that, too, had gone. I settled down for the night in the airport lounge and ate all of the maple sugar candies I had planned to bring back as gifts. Eventually I got home to Warlingham, and was very sad to discover that Auntie Celie had died. I remember Mum mentioning it while I was eating and I had to stop, unable to swallow. She had been out shopping with her dog Biddy and had a heart attack in a shop. I didn't like to think of her dying with strangers.

Travelling over, it felt like time to get settled and face up to making some career plans. Margaret Thatcher's Britain was not ideally suited for this. I received a job offer to work as a recruitment consultant in the Civil Service, but it was withdrawn when the government banned all recruitment. The 80s were a time of mass unemployment, and UB40 sang about the 9.6 per cent unemployment rate in their song "One in Ten". It was also a time of horrendous civil unrest with the miners' strike, the poll tax riots and Clause 28, to name but a few. Watching the news was a daily diet of police on picket lines and soldiers in Northern Ireland. My university friends had moved from the basement flat in Forest Hill, which was so damp their shoes turned green, to a place in Kilburn plagued by dry rot. Still, it was great fun to stay over with them, albeit in a room I had to share with a cat and its litter tray. Elaine had enrolled in training to be a teacher, Jennie was a housing manager, John had a sandwich shop, Carol was contemplating social work, and there were always a couple of others passing through, including Jennie's work colleague Caroline, who kept everyone going with her black forest gateaux. Jennie pointed out an ad in the paper that sought British Airways reservations staff and provided a decent salary and travel benefits. I got the job, located in a large call centre in Kensington known as the West London Terminal. It was not really my forte, but I stuck at it for two years and had discounted travel after 12 months, taking trips to Bermuda, Mexico, Canada, the US and Sri Lanka. I also felt really pleased to arrange discounted flights and a nice hotel for my parents to go to Hong Kong.

During this period I rented a flat in Ladbroke Grove with an old school friend, and I could walk to work through the starkly different environment of North Kensington to wealthy South Kensington. The flat was part of an old Georgian house on Lancaster Road, just off Portobello Road and around the corner from the tube station. The tube was overground and passed inches away from the kitchen window, rattling everything. Below us lived a little old Irish lady who was always complaining that her plants had been stolen from the tiny front garden. One weekend I returned from Clare's to find that there had been a fire in the basement brothel next door, and the residents were very unhappy to have been moved to a high-rise apartment block where footfall was an issue.

Life should have been quite enjoyable, but I found myself clawing my way along just to get through the days. I took a trip to Mexico with Clare and some friends from BA that proved quite stressful because we kept getting robbed. Afterwards, I found myself at the local GP with abdominal pain. She was a warm, friendly American, and I burst into tears as soon as she asked how I was. I really couldn't explain, as this had crept on me unawares, but I said I had suffered from depression before. She confirmed the depression alongside colitis, arming me with medication for both and a certificate for two weeks off work. I don't recall what the antidepressants were, but I do remember an initial sense of great relief that there was an explanation for how I felt. Soon, though, that lightness gave way to miserable, blue feelings. Logically, it should be obvious when a depression is coming on, as I have had them previously, but it doesn't work like that for me. I find myself thinking everything in the world – especially me – is wrong before the penny drops and I can get things in proportion. I slept a lot and tried to make sense of the reasons why to my poor flatmate Mandie, who patiently tried to be reassuring, but I think I left her at a complete loss. To experience utter despair for no good reason is horrible and hard for others to understand.

Over a week or so the drugs took some effect, and getting into a proper sleep pattern provided further relief. Returning to work gave me structure in life again, and I felt pleased to be back with a friend who had noticed my predicament because she had some experience of it herself. She was a no-nonsense Liverpudlian called Suzie, who had a great turn of phrase and a lot of warmth. My confidence had taken a knock, and I worried that I might seem a bit dopey so I kept my head down. Thankfully, I was no longer in the reservations hall, but had moved to a small complaints section to which I felt much better suited. I actually enjoyed dealing with customers' grievances. Time is a healer, but not on its own. I still disliked taking drugs, but I had started to acknowledge an inevitability. In those days it seemed standard practice to prescribe antidepressants for a three-month period only, which left quite a raw adjustment at the end. More recently, eight months or so seems to be the perceived wisdom to avoid relapse and does seem to achieve a gentler recovery. However, it's harder to stop after such a long stretch, in my experience.

Within five or six months, I became aware that I was enjoying life more and seeing friends. Mandie and I went skiing in Aviemore for New Year with some of her Australian friends. It would have been better with more snow and fewer rocks, but we had a laugh. Ladbroke Grove was a great location to experience London, although it could be quite edgy at night. The market stalls on Portobello Road sold antiques and curios, while small record shops played music on good quality sound systems. The Electric Cinema was in its original art deco state, and the Notting Hill Carnival took place on the August bank holiday weekend, although participation was limited because the road was blocked off and the police were stationed in the school opposite. That spring I went on a trip to Sri Lanka with a BA colleague, as we had managed to get free tickets from Paris and just needed to pay 10 per cent of the flight cost from London to Paris. We had time to kill en route and embarked on trying to find the ultimate mousse au chocolat on the streets of Paris. With Skytrain, long-haul travel had opened up a lot, but it was still a time when flights were reasonably empty, so passengers could often sleep on a row of seats. Another colleague at BA had arranged for us to rent a little beachside house on stilts from her aunt in Beruwala. I enjoyed working in travel because of the staff's enthusiasm and because we got to share travellers' tales. On the other hand, a major downside was getting to an amazing place but not having the funds to do it justice. We did travel on a ridiculously crowded bus to the temples at Kandi, which were amazing, despite warnings from our host that unrest amongst the Tamils, a Sri Lankan ethnic group, had started growing on the island. Up until that point I was not aware of the Tamils, but a war between them and the Sinhalese ensued for the next 25 years.

A few days after returning from Sri Lanka, I had a phone call from Clare sounding a bit glum. She had recently moved to Vancouver with her partner David. Months earlier I had taken Mum's Canadian birth certificate to the High Commission in Trafalgar Square to see if I could claim citizenship and, to my surprise, found that I could. Clare had run into financial difficulties in managing a band and decided to apply for her Canadian citizenship in order to move there and get away from it all. She told me that she would be marrying David the following week, as he could not remain in the country otherwise. I had some leave left and said I would come to the wedding, but Clare forbade me from telling anyone. I was not sure why, and I did tell Frances, who was sad not to be part of it. I flew to Vancouver while still getting over jet lag from flying east to Sri Lanka.

Vancouver remains the most beautiful place I have ever seen, nestled between the sea and the mountains. Clare and David had an apartment on the North Shore that seemed incredibly luxurious to me but was actually pretty standard. I slept on a sofa bed they had found in their building's underground garage, and they bought themselves a bed at IKEA. Clare was doing secretarial work, and David had occasional labouring jobs, but they were pretty broke. Clare seemed exhausted. The wedding took place in a friend's house, someone who also had links back to the UK. There was a real sense of welcome and support for newcomers. Clare had booked a minister from the Yellow Pages, and nobody knew what religion he was. It was a lovely day out in the garden with lots of food and wine. A good-natured crowd turned up, and the party went on into the night. "Bette Davis Eyes" played about 100 times. Clare and David went missing soon after the ceremony and turned out to be fast asleep, but they eventually returned to the party.

It was great to catch up with Clare. Because she received her citizenship in Vancouver, she had to go to a ceremony and sing "O Canada," something I had side-stepped when I got mine in the post. I had only met David a couple of times but was pleased to get to know him. I brought him a gold filling in a green set of plaster teeth, as he had been in the process of having treatment at his dentist in Shepherd's Bush before his and Clare's hurried departure, but I think it turned out to be of no use. The three of us spent some time seeing the sights, going to the beaches and up to Deep Cove. The beauty of everything was breathtaking. Clare asked me why I didn't move to Vancouver, too. I didn't stop to think that I was yet again following in her path. I just thought about what a beautiful place it was, that it didn't compare to my dark flat in Ladbroke Grove, and the monotonous work at BA that would never lead to a career for me.

So, I returned home and gave in my notice while I could still get a cheap flight back to Vancouver and air-freight my belongings at 10 per cent of the fare. I didn't worry about any medical implications or even think about them. When I was well I expected to remain well, and when I was depressed, it felt as if I had been born that way and would always be miserable.

7
TWO PSYCHIATRIC HOSPITALS

I enjoyed the flight back to Vancouver, as it felt like an exciting
new beginning, and I think I am drawn to adventures with
surprisingly little worry about how they might turn out. Clare
had spoken to their landlady about a bachelor apartment in their
building, and I inherited the sofa bed until I was able to replace
it. Most furniture tended to be expensive, heavy, old American
colonial-style pieces, so IKEA was great. My first purchase was a
round pine table with four red chairs and a red overhead lamp.
The apartment was a ground-floor room with patio doors that
opened onto shrubs and trees. It had a nice bathroom, a kitchen
area and a walk-in wardrobe. I could forgive the thick, green shag-
pile carpet because it was fitted, and the place had heating and
air-conditioning, too. I loved it. People I had met at the wedding
gave me pots and pans, and a woman from work gave me a ton of
cutlery, as she was getting married and expecting a new set. I still
use some of it.

My first job in Vancouver was a clerical one at BC Tel in their
downtown office, a walk away from the SeaBus that I travelled on
each day. It paid amazingly well, and I found myself making lots
of comparisons with England, where everything seemed scarce
in material terms, but rich in other ways. BC Tel had teams of
engineers, all men except for two women, plus a handful of female
support staff. I often worked with a man called Ron, who amused me
by presenting as hard done by as possible. I had little idea what I was
doing but tried to follow instructions as best as I could.

Everyone seemed sociable and accepting. It was a real melting pot of cultures, and I don't recall any First Nations people who were marginalized at work. There was a draft dodger from the Vietnam War who could never go back to his US home and family because of lasting bitterness towards him from others who had lost sons in the effort. I think he would talk to me about it because I had no direct experience or judgements to make. One of the engineers lived in a Winnebago and would organize trips to go night skiing up on Grouse Mountain before serving his homemade lasagne on board the camper. Another engineer, Craig, took me on skiing trips to Mount Baker over the border in Washington, where the runs went on for miles. He would snowboard on the black runs. My skiing was never that adventurous, but I loved the silence and the beautiful, snowy mountains. It was great having Clare and David living up on the third floor, but we had our own lives and didn't see each other constantly. They often saw British expat friends, while I gravitated towards Canadians.

I hadn't given up on becoming a social worker, so I went into the Women's Resources Centre of the University of British Columbia on Robson Street, where a very dynamic psychologist called Dr Ruth Sigal signed me up as a volunteer peer counsellor to women. At my interview with Ruth, I found myself sharing that I suffered from clinical depression and had started feeling homesick. Sometimes there is one person who has a major impact on your life – for me, that was Ruth. She trained a group of us in client-centred counselling using the work of Carl Rogers and gave us confidence in using our own experience as a resource. I still have my copy of *On Becoming a Person*, and I think it has always informed my practice. We provided a drop-in counselling service, through which we gave one session with advice and signposted other services if needed. Most women wanted to talk about marital issues, money and empty nest syndrome. They tended to be middle aged, and many had long endured their problems in silence, but they drew strength from the female environment to finally open themselves up.

Christmas came and went. I had never seen lights outlining houses, and the boats down by Granville Island had strands on the edges of their sails, too. It was beautiful, and I was struck by how different

Christmas felt without all the usual emotional and historical pressures. Everything seemed lighter somehow. Clare and David gave me a Sony Walkman. They had just come out and were really cool. I bought a cassette of Roxy Music's *Avalon* and listened while I walked on the sea wall. What could be better? I missed my family, and we had a shock when news came that Dad had a heart attack in church. As luck would have it, a husband-and-wife GP pair were sitting behind him during the mass and revived him. The priest rattled through to the end of the mass in quick time, then shouted my dad's name, to which he opened his eyes before heading off in the ambulance. Mum did not tell us any of this until Dad was clearly recovering. It then came to light that he had always had an irregular heartbeat and needed medication thereafter. The church community supported my mum with lifts to the hospital. I had stopped going to church as a teenager, aside from Christmas mass, but I later returned as a parent looking for the positive community and moral compass that I wanted my sons to have. In their early teens we stopped going, as reports of child sexual abuse kept surfacing in waves. Apologies continue to be trotted out, along with messages about learning lessons. All they need to do is obey the laws of the land and use the same law enforcement services as everyone else. In the meantime I bypass the hierarchy and deal directly with God myself.

Apropos of nothing, depression crept up on me again. I recognized the signs more quickly this time. Not eating, not sleeping, trouble concentrating and a sadness that I could feel in my chest. I went to see Dr Rev, a young but very able and thorough doctor with whom Clare had registered. She prescribed antidepressants but also wanted to refer me to a suitable psychiatrist, and she said she would take some time to locate one. Dr Rev also suggested the Women's Resources Centre and did a double take when I said I was a volunteer there. The antidepressants made me very drowsy and, when I went into work, Ron was quite hostile and asked why I had been shooting up. I showed him my prescription bottle, and he couldn't have been nicer, although he insisted on trying to diagnose the situation as either homesickness or lack of nooky. He was protective thereafter, which I greatly appreciated.

An appointment eventually came through for me to see psychiatrist Dr Janine O'Kane. She was British and very pleasant, although I think I was quite wary. She adjusted my medication to Prothiaden, as she hesitated to use newer antidepressants, such as Prozac, preferring to stick to tried-and-tested ones. I seemed to have a lot of weekly appointments with Dr O'Kane, who concluded that I was too fragile for therapy. She would ask me to imagine that my parents were in the room and what I would say, but it would just make me cry. I gave a long life history, and Dr O'Kane took copious notes. She suggested that I was a person who could run well on automatic, in terms of functioning during depression, but perhaps couldn't just let go and have a gin and tonic.

At each session she would ask me if I recalled any high, manic episodes. I don't think I ever really understood the question. I could not identify any wild behaviour, such as excessive shopping, but I think I have probably had mildly high periods before going into a depression. Dr O'Kane would explain that my depression presented as unipolar, but she wondered if it was bipolar or manic depression, which is a less common term now. Over time Dr O'Kane suggested introducing lithium to see if it would help. I was reluctant, but I eventually agreed to take a minimal dose and attend the requisite blood tests to check toxicity levels. Looking back, I'm not sure why I hesitated, but I think I feared that drugs changed me as a person. I can understand why many people choose not to be medicated and lose their high phases, not to mention the drugs' dire impact on the libido.

Regular visits to Dr O'Kane gave me support and a place to review how I was managing and learning to check myself better. By the time the sessions ended, I felt much better and had gained some valuable insight into my mental health. Having high-profile public figures start to share their bipolar diagnoses in recent years has undoubtedly helped normalize things for many people – sufferers and supporters. Back in the 80s I drew scant comfort from hearing about Winston Churchill's so-called black dog of depression.

8
BACK TO BLIGHTY

I soon learnt that the world does not stand still for depression. A different kind of depression – an economic one – was sweeping through Canada and throwing many people out of work, including me. On leaving BC Tel I was very relieved to find that I had worked long enough to qualify for unemployment insurance: 75 per cent of my salary for one year. Initially I enrolled on a government typing course but was hopeless at it, graduating with a dire 17 words per minute. My fellow volunteers at the Women's Resources Centre found themselves unemployed, and these tended to be people who, like me, did the Saturday sessions. One friend, Jacquie, located a government scheme that provided her with seed money to set up a support project for unemployed people in an East Vancouver neighbourhood. We adapted what we had gained at the centre to address the support needs of this diverse group of people, who had either lost their livelihoods or whose battle to find work had just become much harder. We took to cable TV and newspapers for publicity, and it quickly became a well-used resource for people even if we couldn't offer what everyone wanted most, which was work.

Clare and David had moved to a district called South Granville because the North Shore felt quite isolated at that time. Of course, I followed suit and moved into an apartment a few streets away. My new bachelor apartment was in an older, smaller building, and it came with a pink fridge and wooden floors. Clare, David and some friends helped me move. I provided the traditional beer and pizza but forgot the oregano, which I found to make a big difference.

I was closer to friends, to Granville Island and downtown, as well as the beach and Stanley Park. Clare did great barbecues with a little hibachi on the beach at English Bay, and watching the sunset from there was fabulous. Frances brought her children for the summer, and Clare arranged sailing lessons for them. We all went on a beautiful ferry ride to camp on one of the Gulf islands, Galliano, and it was great fun. Frances and I went to see Joan Armatrading in concert, which was a fabulous night out. Things were too good to be true, and I should have realized that a downturn would soon be on its way.

A fellow volunteer at the Women's Resources Centre knew I had struggled with depression, and she told me she was having therapy. We had worked together on making a cable TV series for the WRC, during which time I learnt that I did not excel as a production assistant in charge of the stopwatch, but she made a good interviewer. She knew of an opportunity to have free supervised therapy with a student psychologist attached to the practice she attended. I decided to have an initial consultation and met with the student, who seemed knowledgeable and professional. However, they said that the practice did not work with patients taking medication, as it was not necessary with their support, and they offered an alternative. I had never liked taking medication anyway, so if psychology offered something that psychiatry didn't, I thought I would try it. Responsibly, I went to discuss it with my GP. Dr Rev was on maternity leave, but her locum said it was a good idea to try foregoing my prescription while I had the proper therapeutic support. I cut down and then stopped all medication. In my first couple of appointments with my student psychologist, I gave a background history, to which she made insightful comments. However, I felt there was an emphasis on recovered memory, a method most often used at that time to uncover child sexual abuse. I could only share the experience of the window cleaner, and that didn't seem to satisfy her. I began to feel that I was required to fit into the clinic's agenda rather than them catering their services to meet my needs. During this period I had been doing some work with the Youth Employment Service (YES) also established by Jacquie and linked to a well-respected women's counselling service. They offered me a permanent job with a proper salary and opportunities for training. It was a great offer and exactly what I wanted, but, in the interim, I was going downhill fast.

A strange situation then arose at the YES project when one of the counsellors began to behave erratically and strangely. Clients started to feel nervous around her, and I worried when I noticed that she seemed unwell and hard to reach. She began to bring in herbs and homeopathic remedies for everyone. I raised this with the managers of the centre, and their reaction verged on hostile. They wanted to know, "Did I think she should be on something as terrible as medication?" One day she locked herself in the bathroom and wouldn't respond to us asking her to unlock the door. When we finally got it open, she was flossing her teeth. After some discussion she calmly agreed to go home and contact her GP. I just knew that she wouldn't, as she was in complete crisis. Within a few minutes, someone came in to say that she was turning over dustbins on the surrounding estate. The centre manager finally responded by calling an ambulance to take her to hospital. She was released that evening, and I don't know what happened to her after that. I was really upset and talked to Jacquie about it. The young woman had talked to me about going to see her mother who had a beautiful home. Jacquie paused, then told me that her mother was dead, and this particular counsellor had schizophrenia, but confidentiality agreements had prevented her telling me. I was furious. I said that it was irresponsible to leave me in the dark, as it left me no way to help appropriately. Jacquie told me that the project had been set up to provide employment opportunities to people who had experienced mental health problems. As she talked I realized that that included me without my knowledge. Then, Jacquie said she had similarly maintained confidentiality over my bipolar disorder. This was a nightmare in terms of ethics, safeguarding and responsibilities. I ended my friendship with Jacquie, mainly because I felt betrayed, and I just couldn't cope with anything more at that point.

This episode seemed to trigger a downward spiral. My perceptions and senses started to get distorted. A number of times I went from my apartment to a coffee shop at the end of the road where I would call Clare to say that I couldn't leave, and she would come and get me with varying degrees of patience. I couldn't sleep and phoned the police one night to say that I thought someone was breaking in. In my last interview with the psychologist, I thought she was uncharacteristically wearing heavy makeup, and I must have seemed quite incoherent. She told me that I needed to contact my GP and needed medication. I was only eating peanut butter cookies and, sometimes, just the dough. And, when it came time to start my new job, the person who successfully aced the interview must have borne no relation to the one who turned up on day one and couldn't get beyond lunchtime. David arrived to take me home and was really nice, as were the women with whom I was due to work, but they firmly said I couldn't join them and needed to look after myself. I was shocked, embarrassed and ashamed. I kept going over and over recent events in my mind and coming up with ever more elaborate versions of what had and hadn't happened.

I think Clare probably tried to piece together what had happened and contacted the psychologist's supervisor. Dr O'Kane was on an extended trip to the UK, and Dr Rev remained on maternity leave – a perfect storm. I found myself in the car with Clare and David. They drove me to St Paul's, an old hospital downtown, where they said I would just be staying for the weekend to have a rest. I didn't believe them, but I think I was too numb to protest; plus, I sensed their anxiety. When we arrived, we met a tall grey-suited psychiatrist with a bow tie. While I don't recall anything he said, I took in the air of authority. Clare and David quickly disappeared at his cue, and I found myself being taken to a cubicle and given a gown to put on. When the nurse returned I could see she was holding something behind her back. I wouldn't turn around, so she pushed me forward and injected something that knocked me out. I think it was an antipsychotic drug called haloperidol, otherwise known as the chemical cosh.

My memories of St Paul's are very vague, especially considering I was there for a month. When I did come to, I found my way off the ward and down to the offices, where I demanded to see my notes and find out why I was there. A startled clerk explained that patients couldn't see their notes because they might see something like "SOB" and assume the worst when, really, the acronym just meant "short of breath." I had no idea what she was talking about, and I soon found myself back on the ward with no idea how I got there, although I suspect another injection was involved. The ward was quite noisy and chaotic with lots of comings and goings. I think there were ward meetings, but I may be confusing that with *One Flew Over the Cuckoo's Nest*.

I received a phone call from Mum one day, which was probably quite hard to organize in practical terms. I was too upset to say much, and she said I would be more confident when I came out of hospital. Hard to know how that was going to work, but I could tell she was upset, and I didn't want to make things any worse for either of us. I remember Clare coming to take me out for lunch one day and, when she arrived, I was standing next to a tall, bearded man in black with a large crucifix and a god complex. He was making a lot of noise, so I told him to stop, which he did. Clare thought I was potentially endangering myself by criticizing his behaviour, but I just saw him as a fellow patient. I wasn't getting better, and Clare explained that the psychiatrist had diagnosed me as having a personality disorder and not bipolar, so they did not prescribe me any lithium. Even in my groggy state, this sounded like bad news. By then, Dr O'Kane had returned to Vancouver, but she had no jurisdiction in St Paul's. I was given leave to spend a weekend at home as a means of rehabilitation, and I just didn't go back. Nobody seemed to follow it up.

Someone made an appointment for me to see Dr O'Kane at Shaughnessy Hospital, and she asked that I bring a change of clothes. I went with Clare, and I probably acted quite erratically in my discussion with Dr O'Kane. I remember her asking why I had brought my bag if I didn't want to go to hospital, and I replied, "Because you asked me to." Dr O'Kane said that I had done nothing wrong, but she feared that I would do something silly if I wasn't admitted under a section. Clare had to sign the forms, and I think that must have been terrible for her. I feel deeply sad to think about it now.

After St Paul's, Shaughnessy Hospital felt light, bright and even friendly, but some of my optimism may have stemmed from the lithium that I had started taking again. The staff wheeled around a large trolley full of freshly laundered cotton pyjamas and dressing gowns from which we could choose, and we could pick the kind of food we wanted at the hospital's restaurant. Those things really mattered to me at a time when I had little control over my life.

Dr O'Kane explained that, because I had previously been on a low dose of lithium, stopping it had resulted in a rapid crash. It took time to get well, and the first weeks were difficult. At one point I got my own room because I made a lot of noise at night, disturbing the rest of the ward. When my locum GP made a visit, I heard one of the nurses telling her that I was difficult and noisy. I do recall one occasion when four nurses wrestled me on to my bed, but I don't know what led to this. My memories are sketchy, so, in that sense, those were a lost couple of months. I do vividly recall sitting in the restaurant on one occasion, eating at a table with another patient, and then suddenly deciding that I was going to climb out of the window. We were on the ground floor. I didn't get far before a nurse tugged on my pyjamas and gave me an injection in the thigh. There must have been other instances like this that I cannot recall, and I obviously needed the hospital to keep me safe, but losing my freedom and being so vulnerable is still hard to think about.

Some weeks later Dr Rev visited and said I had been badly behaved, according to reports. Mad or bad? This time I defended myself, somewhat exasperatedly, by saying that I was ill, and she accepted that, saying she wished her locum had taken more time before advising me to stop my medication. Some friends started to visit, and that was important, because it was hard to know how I would be perceived as a mental patient when I eventually re-joined the outside world. Jacquie came and brought a copy of *The New Yorker*, which she knew I liked. We had been really good friends, and she said she had received a lot of criticism for how she had dealt with things.

Although she was talented, I think she lacked experience and put too much of her focus on funding. I just wanted to move on, and she seemed to want the same.

As I came to the end of my stay in hospital I had a last appointment with Dr O'Kane, whose parting advice was not to think too much about my aunt. I got another lithium prescription to continue to stabilize my mood swings in the long term, and they gave me no other drugs. Lithium is a natural element, but it's also potentially toxic, so I needed regular blood tests to monitor the level of it in my system. Some patients in the hospital told me that they had been taking it for decades.

I planned a trip home to the UK for Christmas. Sadly, I had missed John's wedding, but my parents were celebrating their ruby wedding anniversary on New Year's Day in 1984, so I could be there for that. I got myself a return ticket because I didn't want future plans to be determined solely by my hospitalization. Arriving at Heathrow where Mum and Anthony were waiting felt unreal, and I had a huge sense of relief as I always did when returning home. I also had a sense of failure and awkwardness – the return of the mental patient. Thankfully, those thoughts did not persist for long. I comfortably settled into life in my parents' cottage, watching *Dallas* and having a sherry with Mum, going for walks and making trips to London, plus having dinner at Julie's with her new husband Paul. Actually, I had forgotten about the dinner invitation, and I ate before I arrived but didn't like to say. Julie was very concerned about my appetite, as well as my verdict on her cooking. I ate and slept well, losing the hospital paleness, and I started being able to enjoy living in the moment. It was good to have privacy after hospital life.

Frances made a lovely celebratory meal for the 40th wedding anniversary with lots of ruby-coloured dishes, and everyone was there apart from Clare and David. I was conscious of people looking at me and wondering about me, but this was my tribe, and I felt I belonged. Nonetheless, I needed to return to Vancouver and decide whether to stay or go; otherwise, it would feel like I had unfinished business and just gave up. I think my family was surprised that I planned to return.

Despite all of the mental health issues I had experienced there, I really liked Vancouver, its way of life and its people.

After a month in England, I returned to my tiny apartment on West 11th Avenue and caught up with friends. I am not sure my landlord was pleased I came back, as he had had to endure my pacing on the wooden floor all night, but he was welcoming. I can't recall how it came about, but I was reinstated in my job at BC Tel. They didn't need to take me back, especially as I was pretty rubbish at the job, so I felt grateful. It was great to be accepted without any stigma. This proved to be a time of introspection for me, and I went for many walks on the beach at English Bay and around Stanley Park. I knew that I had to commit to Canada or England, as I needed to build a career. Now that I felt better, it seemed possible.

After a few months, I made the decision to return to my roots in the UK, where family really mattered. I longed for shop assistants to be rude to me, and I couldn't live on scenery, as much as I loved it. Before I left, Craig persuaded me to go water skiing in Deep Cove because I would never get the chance in England. So, I put on a cold wetsuit, pulled myself up on my first try and skied slowly round the cove. An otter popped its head up nearby, and I signalled to Craig to pull in. As I am virtually a non-swimmer, it was amazing and a lovely memory to have.

Ron and the BC Tel crowd took me to a piano bar in the West End for a goodbye drink. Clare and David took me out to dinner on Granville Island at Bridges, and I knew there was going to be a lot of food that I would miss. I had a degree of ambivalence about my decision, but it came down to where I had the strongest sense of belonging. I booked a cheap single flight from Seattle on Hawaiian Airlines, and a friend from the Women's Resources Centre drove me down there. Because it was Hawaiian's inaugural flight to London, the staff kept putting orchid necklaces around our necks and serving champagne constantly with a forced jollity. It was horrible. I was glad to land at Heathrow and head back to Warlingham, where I was to stay for the next six months. Canada quickly seemed a distant memory – that is, until Clare wrote to me saying she had told Anthony's wife about my bipolar disorder in case of genetic inheritance implications for his children. It was too soon, and it needed to come from me. I felt like some sort of alien species with my information being hijacked. Mum could see I was upset, and she phoned Clare about it. Disability is complex in terms of information and how it is handled.

9
PUTTING DOWN ROOTS

Mum and Dad had settled into retirement in the village of
Warlingham, and Nestle had given Dad a greenhouse. They didn't
pay well but they were good on pensions, watches at 25 years and
otherwise marking special occasions. His parting after 40 years of
service had been celebrated with a dinner at a London hotel from
whence Mum returned in high dudgeon. In a speech it was noted
that Dad was offered his manager's job when he retired, but he
turned it down because he wanted to spend more time with his
family. Mum was hearing this for the first time, and aside from the
financial aspect and unilateral decision-making, she was exasperated
that he never had any confidence in himself. Mum insisted that
Dad have an allotment so he didn't invade her space in the cottage.
He wasn't really a gardener, but he enjoyed the digging and the
company of the other allotment holders. I don't think I ever saw
any produce. Mum had joined an art class that met most weeks,
apart from when the teacher would suddenly take off to the South
of France in his battered caravan. They probably thought their
parenting days were over, but I loved being an only child at 29.

Once I had caught up with friends, my priority was to get my
social work career underway. Margaret Thatcher had intervened in
my life again by changing the immigration rules. Because I had lived
outside the UK for more than three years, I was classed as an overseas
student with no access to funds for my social work training. Instead, I
approached the local authority for related unqualified work and was
hired to work in a children's home as a residential social worker.

On day one I arrived at eight in the morning and was met by a handsome young Asian man in a smoke-filled office. Everyone smoked, including the kids. I noticed that he was wearing a gold ring and assumed he was married. He later told me that he had borrowed a comb from one of the kids, as he had been sleeping in and felt too scruffy to impress. It was a bit of a thunderbolt moment, and Joel remains my life partner.

The children's home looked like all the houses on the surrounding estate, where every other household seemed to have a rottweiler. There was an uneasy relationship between the home and local community, who saw it as a source of trouble. Sometimes it was, but sometimes the local environment posed challenges, too. Some nights a black car with music blaring would drive up without lights, and mostly young children would be seen scurrying to it as if it was an ice cream van. However, they ran to the vehicle to get drugs, most often for their parents. Glue sniffing was the cheaper choice for some of our kids, who always denied it but showed the signs. Another new danger lurked in the form of HIV/AIDS, which had everyone thinking about their sexual health, past and present. It posed yet another risk for our vulnerable kids, who were so easily exploited by the paedophile rings that society had finally begun to acknowledge. On a positive note I did a weekend shift when the first Live Aid concert aired, and we all enjoyed it at a considerable volume on the one and only rented TV.

When I started, most of the eight residents were boys in their late teens who had been in care for many years. One young boy would come from boarding school for his holidays, and the neighbours would come knocking before he arrived to say that they didn't want him there, as they had enough problems on the estate. He was exuberant, mischievous, and had a talent to create mayhem out of nothing. It was hard not to have a soft spot for him, especially when he brought recruits to the door who he thought should be in care as well. Over time girls came into the home, and then younger siblings for whom there was no space in foster care joined us so that they could remain with their brothers and sisters. For a time, there was even a parrot called Brian, but one of the care staff liberated him and took him home after he was found with a lit cigarette in his beak. I had a sense of deja vu.

The purpose of the home changed from a long-stay institution to a short-stay unit in which children had care plans to move on. Even with a timeline, though, this process could still take several years. They were all decent kids who had been through unimaginable horrors and were still replaying their early life experiences without the benefit of therapy. We tried to have smooth handovers, and we took copious notes in a day book, but being cared for by shift workers was far from ideal. All of the unfinished courses of antibiotics were testimony to that. Children often absconded at night and had to be reported to the police, but it was sometimes impossible for those on shift to give a description if they had never seen them. We received the suitcase of a lad called Cosmo three times in the space of a month, but never did get to meet him. One evening I said goodbye to a young man who had dressed up to go to a party. Five minutes later a policeman handed him over and said, "We've got one of yours." I protested, but they said they would be looking for him at midnight anyway, so he might as well come back now. The young man had made the mistake of giving another boy's name who had been reported as missing. Parents seemed to think we were much too soft and often asked why we didn't lock them into the house.

Routine and predictability were probably the only useful strategies available to give a sense of security. I think my best qualification was having grown up in a large household where I learnt to attune myself to moods, crises and relationships, taking defensive action where needed. My biggest shortcoming was in catering, as we had to cook frozen food that was delivered to us by lorry. Sausages were always put next to my name on the rota, as my colleagues felt I couldn't go wrong – but they were mistaken. I used to hide enormous containers of orange squash that we called Agent Orange because it made everyone hyper very quickly. I soon had the role of attending juvenile court because I was deemed to have the right speaking voice for it and didn't find it intimidating. I also attended Child Guidance, now Child and Adolescent Mental Health Services, at times. The perceived wisdom, for good reasons, was that children should not commence therapy unless they were in a stable and permanent living situation. Our children seldom seemed to be, so occasionally a consultation would be offered with a child psychiatrist and then shared with the staff group. I would see a lovely Italian man to discuss managing behaviour, but it was hard to understand a lot of what he was saying, as he had a heavy accent. I would arrive back to my expectant colleagues and talk about parent figures providing good endings. "But what do we do?" they would say as their faces fell over listening to what they thought was psychobabble.

One summer I saw the Italian psychiatrist on a fortnightly basis about a deeply troubled girl. She had been sexually abused and exploited in many ways, and she had only her deep anger and spirit to keep her going. I had to take her to the High Court in the Strand, which is a very forbidding place, to meet the judge who would decide her future. She was frightened, and on the way back to Charing Cross, she screamed wildly with the noise of the traffic along the road. I could only hold her hand to keep her safe. In time she had to move on to a more secure environment, and the psychiatrist offered me a session to look at the impact her case had on me, which was really kind, unexpected and professional. He probably identified a vulnerability in me. It was hard work to be around children and young people who could be unpredictable and spark each other into extreme behaviour. We had a trainer who sometimes came when we were really under pressure. She would talk about encouraging the children to regress and have some of the early childhood experiences that they had missed. It made perfect sense, but I recall an indignant Irish man saying, "So a teenager is coming at me with a machete, and I should be making him sloppy nursery food?" We did keep an arsenal of confiscated weapons that we handed over to the police every year. When possible, I would sometimes play games with the kids from my childhood like murder in the dark, which would have the toughest lads giggling like small children and accepting a light touch that they never would normally.

After six months I was asked to apply for a permanent post, which involved completing a medical questionnaire. I had to be honest and face the possibility that I would not be deemed suitable with my mental health history. Perhaps it would apply to all jobs. I talked to Frances about it, and she said she knew of a psychiatrist who might be able to advise me. I contacted him and made an appointment, but he said I had to go to my GP and get a referral. I saw a locum GP and explained the situation while she became red-faced and very angry. She said that I was trying to manipulate the system. Because I did not know what she meant or why she seemed so hostile, I kept quiet and, after glaring at me, she said she would make the referral but not happily. I was not sure why she had such an apparently low opinion of me, as we had never met before, but I didn't think any further about it. I saw the psychiatrist, who I think was quite senior. He took a look at my history and was insightful. He said he felt it would be bad luck if I didn't get the job on the basis of my bipolar disorder, as I was managing it well and had been doing the job for six months. His view seemed realistic and gave me confidence. On the morning of the medical, I nevertheless felt sick. Mum asked a friend if he could drive me to Croydon, which he kindly did. The meeting was quite short and, after asking a few questions, the medical adviser basically said that I had been ill and was now better. She did not have an issue. I came out into the corridor, took the lid off a large black bin and was sick into it. I replaced the lid and left thinking that I had just left a horrible mess for someone to clear up. My anxiety was all about my identity and whether the manic-depressive label would be my defining characteristic. My sense of relief was huge, and I was delighted to sign my contract. I rapidly went from residential social worker to senior residential social worker, then assistant officer-in-charge.

Once I had secured a permanent job, I went flat hunting. In the mid-80s a mortgage was cheaper than renting, and I located a studio flat in South Croydon above a gun shop. The market was moving rapidly, and I went with Dad to a number of building societies to seek a mortgage. I don't think they were keen on single women, but finally we found a young female manager at the Yorkshire Building Society who agreed to lend over 35 years and said she thought it was likely I would increase my earnings with promotion. I got back to the seller who said the flat had gone, but he had a one-bedroom property in the same renovated building. We rushed round to see it, and it was much nicer. Dad offered to lend me the extra money toward the deposit, and we secured it. I think Mum and Dad must have been very relieved that I had established my independence, as they could not have predicted this when I had so recently been in hospital in Canada. I know they had considered changing their wills in case I was not able to earn a living. The flat was roomy with large sash windows that looked down onto the busy high street with lots of restaurants. Late at night we could hear the Chinese chefs and waiters gambling.

My partner moved in, and life was too busy to dwell on my mental health. I told him about it, but he never seemed particularly interested, although I knew he had a knowledge of mental health. Joel helped me finally pass my driving test on the fifth attempt, and I drove several old £50 bangers that he bought. We went to Scotland in an Austin Allegro that only had suspension on one side. While there we fished in Loch Fine and caught nothing, although everyone around us were pulling in fish and putting them straight onto barbecues. They offered us different types of fly as bait to no avail, and I think Joel lost interest in fishing for good after that. When Joel bought an automatic Fiat, it changed driving completely. Three pedals had never worked for me, and now I was able to look through the windscreen without looking down at my feet. The whole world was safer.

When I registered with the local GP, I was referred to psychiatric services at Mayday Hospital to have my lithium and general well-being monitored. The service operated from a very grungy temporary building, but the psychiatrist was good. We always had a brief talk, and occasionally I had antidepressants prescribed in addition to the lithium if my mood was particularly low. Sometimes she would disagree with me and say that it was just life, there were legitimate reasons why I might feel depressed, and I could manage without antidepressants. It was really useful feedback because I was getting to know my disorder better, and I found her very reliable. My bipolar disorder is hard to predict because the brief manic phases go largely unnoticed by me until the depression sets in and I realize that I am in an episode. This can be in response to a life event or stress, or it can happen for no apparent reason at all. I function reasonably well when I am depressed and keep my expectations quite realistic after years of practice and structure in my life. I used to feel emotional about it until I learnt to keep in mind my view that the illness is a chemical problem in the brain and therefore physical. That makes it sound easier than it is.

I spent several years at the children's home and lived through some extraordinary experiences with the benefit of a close, supportive staff, which included some great characters and some not-so-great ones. You needed to be able to trust who you were on shift with, and I was mostly with a young man who the kids respected as a role model. At age 16 he had fought in the Falklands War, joining the combat on his first voyage in a submarine. He also had impressive tattoos and the sort of streaks in his hair that they all wanted. Sometimes Crystal Palace Football Club would give us free tickets, and I remember taking the kids to a game with Millwall, who had a terribly violent and racist reputation in the 80s. When Palace scored everyone jumped up, only to find the stands hadn't been divided by team, so everyone had to cover up their tattoos and sit quietly before we snuck out early. A mounted police horse reared up as we went through the gate.

At the home we were supposed to have three on shift, but if it meant having an agency worker, we would decline, as it was often more trouble than it was worth. One weekend we took the kids camping overnight somewhere in Sussex. We were on our final warning half an hour after arriving at the campsite, but everyone settled down. We had a completely sleepless night before a barbecued breakfast and our return home. I thought it was awful, but for months and years afterwards, teenagers would come back and say, "Do you remember when we went camping?" Joel had moved to an assessment centre and arranged to do his formal social work training. He applied to Croydon College, simply on the basis that it was local, and he found himself on a highly psychodynamic course that he thought ridiculous and didn't fit with his pragmatic, down-to-earth approach.

Everyone was in therapy, and everyone kept making disclosures about themselves. I would have loved it. I thought I would need to be the breadwinner during this period, but I was seconded by the local authority to do my training at Bromley College on full pay.

Sadly, just beforehand, my mum passed away. She had been diagnosed with high blood pressure, but her GP advised her to make a planned trip to Vancouver with Dad to see Clare's new baby and have treatment on her return. She applied for her own Canadian passport for the trip, having previously travelled on my dad's British one. They had a great time and were able to be at the christening. When they got back I could see that Mum was struggling, and the last straw was when her oven blew up and burnt the Christmas cake to a crisp. Mum and Dad had Christmas dinner with us at the flat around a tiny table. She said that she had cooked the Christmas dinner for the previous 44 years and, although it was nicely cooked by Joel, it felt very odd for her. The following month Mum had a mini stroke that left her confused for a short time. She told the GP that she was not going to hospital under any circumstances, but she stayed in bed and took aspirin. When I went to see her, she said she'd had her warning. She phoned friends to let them know. I asked if I could call Clare, but she firmly said no. Anthony's wife Rosemary had been to visit with their youngest child, and Mum said he was looking at her curiously through the spindles on her lovely carved Indian bed. I think she was saying that she didn't want to be pitied. I made dinner for my Dad, and Mum asked for some. She rallied a bit, but early the next morning I had a call from the Italian parish priest saying, "Come now." I couldn't get an answer as to whether she was still alive, and I rushed there on the bus. Before leaving I tried to contact Frances and left a message with her daughter to call her. It didn't occur to me that her daughter would probably know what was happening and was left desperately upset at home on her own. My dad had, of course, called the priest before he called the doctor, but she would have wanted that. Mum had passed away bravely at 72. She always said she didn't want to linger beyond her four score and ten years. I don't think she wanted to be disabled or a burden. I admired her resolve, but I wished she had stayed longer. I remember going up to the bedroom to see her and realizing that, once we're dead, there really is nothing left.

Dad seemed to be in shock for a long time. The funeral was attended by family, friends and neighbours. I remember Auntie Mollie holding my hand by the graveside. Clare came from Canada with her baby for the funeral and stayed with Dad for six weeks. They pushed the pram to the cemetery every day, and Clare later commented that her son had spent an extraordinary proportion of his young life in a graveyard. Dad had bought Mum a new anorak for a birthday that she didn't reach, and having it at home seemed to trouble him. Clare and I took it back to Allders, where a pedantic manager kept quizzing us about why we were returning it and explaining in great detail that there was a sale on that affected the amount of the refund. We didn't care about the money, and it seemed extraordinary that she was so devoid of empathy when we were clearly grieving. It made us angry, but then again, so did everything. After two weeks off work, I returned but struggled to manage the grief and anger that welled up when I least expected it. I remember walking in the door and finding staff complaining that one young boy couldn't go to school because he had hidden his trousers. My usual calmness deserted me. I was coming from a major life event and this was all about clothes. I put my face close to the boy and barked at him to get his trousers, which he did instantly. That outburst told me that I was not in control, and I arranged to see the psychiatrist for a new prescription. I probably didn't actually need it, as there is a difference between depression and genuine grief, but I didn't want to experience either. I didn't take any more time off work because I wanted to keep busy, however beneficial grieving might have been. It was a very painful time.

A few months later I started college. Leaving the children's home was a bit sad, but I didn't miss the shift work that included sleeping there at night alone or the shock waves that would go through my knees when an incident occured. The course was not a particularly good one, and the London Borough of Lambeth had withdrawn from the programme, as it was not sufficiently anti-discriminatory. We were an almost all-white student group, which felt very strange and disadvantaged us. The Children Act 1989 had just passed, which divided responsibilities for child welfare between parents, local authorities, courts and other agencies. However, it was not yet fully in use, so we had no case law to study other than the previous childcare acts, so the timing was unfortunate. It was a radical piece of legislation that changed everything.

We were all required to spend a residential week in winter at a dreary hotel in Bournemouth that served everything with cress. The most memorable event, aside from discovering MTV on the hotel TV, was being taught Morris dancing one evening by one of the Kent students who went on to become a Labour Member of Parliament in the 1997 landslide election and then a Minister for Agriculture. One of my fellow students contacted him after seeing him on television, and a group of us had dinner with him at the House of Commons. The food was really good and cost next to nothing. Seeing my hero Barbara Castle holding court in the Pugin Room was wonderful.

My two years at college passed quickly with social work placements and a great deal of written work. There were opportunities to try out working with different client groups, although I was committed to children and families. I spent several months at an agency in Clapham Junction working with adults and making meticulous process recordings that taught us so much. My main concern, however, was a student who kept putting up her hand for every case at allocation, then putting them in her drawer. I tried to talk to her about it, but she would laugh it off. Eventually her tutor wrestled her drawer open and took out 19 untouched referrals. I'm not sure what the issue was, but I don't think it went well for her.

In a generic locality setting, I had a service user with long-standing mental health problems, and it confirmed to me that I would not want to choose this client group, as there could be a danger of over-identification. I found myself incandescent after a phone call with her psychiatrist, who called her a silly old woman, and a meeting with her mother who described her as the family tragedy. On a visit to her flat, I encountered a man under a sheet on the sofa who rose up and slowly but extravagantly introduced himself. I later found that he was a hospital resident who was on licence to the Home Office, having murdered his wife and subsequently undergoing a lobotomy. He should not have been there, and it was decided that I should not be meeting him as a student. The policy seemed less clear for my client. Brain surgery is not a precise science, and I don't know why more effort is not made to understand it. Hearts seem to trump everything. Mental illness features prominently in all forms of social work, but much is undiagnosed, untreated and located out in the community. I have rarely found that having bipolar disorder has given me any additional insight as a social worker, but I think it has always given me respect for people who are struggling.

10
BECOMING A PARENT

Once I had my qualification, I took a job with the Croydon family placement team. It was hoped that I would go back into residential work, where qualified staff were badly needed, but we were thinking about starting a family, and I wanted a safer and more structured job. The team worked in a lovely Georgian building with three large desks to a room and parking that we took for granted at the time. Initially I found it incredibly dull to be sitting at a desk and reading reports without the buzz of the unexpected, as every day had been unpredictable in the children's home. The stresses of my new job were of a different kind, though, and I would carry knowledge of a lot of disturbing cases of abuse in my head over the months that it took to place children in new families. I worked in a small team and learnt a great deal more than I had at college. Those colleagues, most of whom are retired, are now my book group. We try to steer away from interpreting every book through the eyes of social workers, particularly for the sake of the one group member who is a hairdresser and keeps us grounded.

The housing market in the late 80s was wild and unpredictable. Clare and David moved back to the UK and found themselves mired in negative equity as the interest rate climbed to 15 per cent. During a brief upward blip in the market, I sold the flat for more than twice what I paid for it, and we made a smart move to a three-bed semi in Kenley that had been heavily discounted. I was pleased to be moving to a freehold house, as leaseholds can be tricky. One winter, snow on the roof had leaked into our flat and, although we were not the top flat, there was a section of flat roof above us. It was during the 1987 storm when large swathes of roofs and trees came down, but I managed to find builders to mend the roof. They completed it quickly, but when I approached the other residents about sharing the bill, the owner of the gun shop refused because he had seen no evidence of the scaffold for which I had claimed. I really dislike situations like this and I became very anxious, particularly when the builders said they could always come and take their tiles off if I didn't pay. I dreaded picking up the phone, but eventually the leaseholder sent his builder to inspect the roof. He said they had done a good job and risking themselves without a scaffold was up to them, so they got paid. I felt relieved, as the situation was dominating my thoughts all the time. I tend to have similar anxieties about garage personnel and estate agents. The one who sold the flat was just down the road, and we ended up with two people having a slight bidding war. The agent tried to persuade me that the young woman was more reliable but had a strict financial limit, while he knew nothing about the potential male buyer. I said that as long as the man could pay, he seemed fine to me. Later I popped in to see the agent and found the young woman sitting on his desk. There are so many ways to be ripped off.

On moving day a large number of men with a huge van arrived. They had been undercut on another job and given us as consolation. They removed the sash windows to lower the furniture onto the street and, at the other end, they even unpacked the books onto the bookshelves. Dad, Frances and her children came round and sat out in the garden with nothing needing to be done. I would have happily settled for a two-bedroom character cottage, but Joel was more savvy financially, and it was a good move. In the small front garden of our new home was a magnificent magnolia tree, but it was huge and its branches were knocking on the windows. Our neighbour suggested a tree surgeon but my Dad took it upon himself to massacre the poor thing, and I don't think Joel ever forgave him.

We settled in well, but some months later I began to feel depressed for no reason that I could discern at the time, although I now realize that moving could have been the cause. I went to our new GP surgery and saw a rather shrill doctor who asked me what I was doing about all this. I said I was expecting antidepressants, and she persisted in saying, "But what are you doing about it?" She felt I needed to have therapy from her husband, who was an elderly psychologist. I had an appointment with him at her house but found no connection with his Jungian approach. It just felt odd, and it was also going to be expensive. I left feeling a bit sorry for him, as he was likely to incur the wrath of his wife, who was clearly trying to drum up business for him. I made an appointment with a different GP and explained what had happened. He was quite displeased and said that research had shown that therapy was of no use with bipolar disorder. Instead, he referred me to a new psychiatrist in Purley at a joyless building with tiny rooms.

My new psychiatrist was mostly silent. He would make a visual appraisal as I entered the room, then avoid all eye contact. Somehow he seemed to make the right assessment very quickly and with minimum fuss. One day he was unusually running late, and there were two other women in the snug waiting room. We talked about how he was almost always on time because he didn't speak. One woman said she had wondered about wishing him a Happy Christmas but thought it might be the wrong religion. We laughed, and she said thoughtfully that she wished the public could see us as we are... just normal.

After a year or so, I said that I wanted to stop all medication and try for a baby. The psychiatrist said that, in that case, he would not need to see me again because he would not need to monitor my medication. I left while trying to absorb what seemed like amazingly warped logic. I was very worried about whether I would manage motherhood given Auntie Celie's challenging experiences, and I wondered what would happen to me without medication. I feared passing on my genetic legacy, never mind global warming and the rest of the world's issues. My partner was much more confident than I was, but we wanted a family. I sent a handwritten letter to the psychiatrist explaining that I still needed help to manage life without medication from someone who could recognize the signs if

I was becoming unwell. I needed support with having a baby, too. It seemed obvious to me, but I tried to put it diplomatically, as I sensed he could be easily offended if criticized. To my relief, he offered me an appointment and did see me regularly throughout my pregnancy. He advised that someone would need to be with me all the time during the first week after the birth in case of puerperal psychosis or acute postnatal depression. He organized for me to start medication after the birth, as I did not feel confident to be without it, although he recommended breastfeeding for bonding if I felt able to take the risk. We built more of a rapport during this time, and he even talked a bit about his family.

During pregnancy I remained well, and I think the hormonal changes helped my mood. I became absolutely enormous, and I felt concerned about how this might affect the people I worked with who could not have children of their own. My GP organized my antenatal care, and I noticed that the brown envelope that held my medical notes had a large, orange sticker on it. He then told me that, at 34, I was not a spring chicken, which seemed less than helpful, but it just made me laugh. At that time it was pretty elderly for a primigravida, but I had to wait until I was as sure as I could be that I could manage parenthood.

After a very long labour, our son Ben was born safely but with a head injury from forceps, and he needed light therapy for jaundice. When I woke up on the ward, I found myself looking at an empty cot. A nurse came by and said that I had been so tired that they had given Ben a bottle for me, and he was so beautiful that they were really enjoying him. I felt quite bewildered, as though he had been taken away from me. I must have done something wrong and probably shouldn't have said that I suffered from bipolar disorder, but I did because I wanted to protect Ben in case there was any problem. He was returned to me but had to stay under the lamps in his cot. I was relieved when Joel got back, as I was feeling lost. We had strict instructions that Ben could not be picked up, and no visitors were to hold him, either. A lot of people came along at the same time: Dad; Rosemary, who popped his first toy in his cot; Julie with gladioli; Clare and David plus their children; and Frances and her family. A very officious nurse rounded them up and told them they had to come in separately, taking turns. Dad picked up Ben and told the nurse that he knew how to hold a baby. It was a lovely welcome. Joel's family came the next day, which was nice, but I was sad not to have Mum. The following day I remember defiantly picking Ben up and putting him in bed with me, strictly against orders. A new nurse came on duty and smiled, saying, "You are getting to know your baby." She made such a difference.

At home everything seemed magical, and I just wanted to look at Ben. When everything was peaceful I put him in his Moses basket next to the bed and felt a rush of emotion as I looked down at him. I think that was bonding, something I felt all of the time with my second son Oliver, as I had become more confident and less fearful as a mother. When Joel came to bed, he wanted to move Ben in case I trod on him in the night, but I was adamant that he was not going anywhere. It was amazing how quickly the time went on, changing nappies and giving bottles. I had signed up to attend a National Childbirth Trust (NCT) class and received a call from a rather forthright woman, who insisted I come to her house the following day. I explained that I had not managed to get dressed all week, never mind leaving the house, but I found myself agreeing. The following morning I drove round the corner to her house and carried Ben down the stairs in his car seat – amazingly exhausting. The NCT coordinator opened the door and said that all the group were still pregnant, so perhaps we wouldn't mention difficult births. That was a challenge, as I think women need to talk to each other about birth in order to get over it. They were very nice women and naturally curious, but I sidestepped a lot of their questions. In the months and years to come, we would meet up and share our experiences of giving birth. I had a slight dilemma when someone said she didn't know what a social worker might think, and I had to share that I was one, then made a note to myself always to pre-empt that situation. Other friends and work colleagues had babies around the same time, so it did feel a bit like joining a club, as we all had the same focus on things like *Teletubbies* and snowsuits, which was probably really boring to anyone else. Ben and, later, his brother, were baptized at the church where I had attended mass for much of my childhood. Frances helped to arrange this with the priest she knew, as Joel and I were not married. By the time we got to Oliver, he did ask if we intended to get married. As a child of the 70s, I had never wanted a legal relationship, although last year we had a civil partnership ceremony during the COVID-19 lockdown with our boys as witnesses, simply to protect our finances. It was quite jolly with a cup of tea afterwards, and having it at that time was the perfect excuse to avoid a big spectacle. Otherwise, there are not many good things to say about a pandemic.

I returned to work after maternity leave, which I had enjoyed very much, and found it quite an adjustment. Financially, I needed to work, but I also thought I would be a better working mother than a stay-at-home one, as the latter could make me isolated or depressed. I worried about attachment and whether my parenting was good enough. When Ben was three, Oliver was born. It was another long labour, and the midwife was rushed off her feet when my blood pressure could not be brought under control. The consultant was never to be found, and he did not inspire confidence when located. When he broke my membrane, he didn't seem to realize he would get drenched while sitting on my bed. Plus, the stitches he used were not dissolving ones. After considerable discomfort, I managed to get them taken out by an experienced district nurse at the GP surgery, and she said the stitches were in strange places and some didn't serve any purpose. I did wonder if the consultant was actually qualified.

Joel and Ben visited the hospital, and Ben carried a bunch of long-stemmed flowers down the ward like a spear that he whacked down on the bed. Very angry with me and Joel, Ben eventually liked his brother, although it took years before he stopped asking why he had to come. I was reminded of John's birth and the fuss made of him while my jealousy knew no bounds. I found a very good childminder named Bernie, who lived close by with children of a similar age. She worked with us for years when both of our children were young, and we still remain friends. That gave me a lot of reassurance when I was at work, as I had complete faith in her. When I used to collect the boys, Oliver would often have ribbons in his hair and elaborately draped shawls that the Bernie's daughters had arranged. They all went on to the same school, and one of Bernie's daughters was in Ben's class. One day a week Joel's parents, who also had two of his brothers living with them, had the boys, and they were spoilt to bits. They would always help in an emergency, and we very often went to their house for chicken curry on a Saturday.

When they were between house moves, Joel's parents stayed with us for a while, and his mum asked me if I stayed up to watch the children while they slept. I explained that I needed to sleep and go to work. She said she always had people to watch the children through the night in India. Joel's parents had lived very different lives as wealthy, privileged Anglo-Indians who then came to the UK in the early 60s with nothing. They found they were no longer accepted in India because their forebears had intermarried with the British in the time of the Raj and, although they had British passports, western clothes and regarded themselves as British, they were seen as Indian in the UK. It was a complex history to manage. They had no Indian languages, and they learnt to cook Indian food in England. Through hard work they brought up four boys and bought a house. They were practicing Catholics, and I think that helped their sense of belonging. Our support network was good. We had the same health visitor who was helpful both times and noticed that Oliver had a squint. Tiny, gold, John Lennon-style glasses were prescribed from the age of eight months, and they made him a celebrity on the playground at Ben's school. Ben suffered from asthma as a baby and still does, which was quite a learning curve. There was no history of asthma in either family, and Joel's mother told me emphatically that there was no asthma in India. We also had to deal with the controversy of the MMR vaccine and autism when Oliver was due to have it. There was a growing awareness of autism around that time, and some incorrectly linked it to the immunization. I knew how dangerous childhood illnesses could be, so we went ahead with it. However, we chose the option of two spaced-out jabs so that his immature immune system might manage it more easily. I was always watchful for clear signs of autism and, later on, bipolar disorder, but thankfully there has not been anything significant.

I usually noticed the early signs of my own depression, but sometimes Joel would prompt me to get help if I was seeming blank or inexplicably tearful. Work helped to keep me grounded, and I very rarely took a day off sick. My team were supportive and child-friendly, as many of them either had young families or understood the demands. An important source of support for me were Julie's parents, and I would drop by when I could. Julie's mum would ask me about my mental health, and that felt comforting. They were always good company, and I would feel all the warmth from my childhood visits. One day I had put a tint on my hair to hide the grey that was appearing. Julie's mum had famously thick auburn hair that she kept immaculately. She explained her regime for colouring that I still use to this day, and as I was leaving she emphasized, "Not maroon."

All of my time outside work was with the children, and that was really all that seemed important. I probably was slightly overprotective as a social worker, but Joel was more so. I think I would have been far less confident had I been a younger parent less at ease with managing her bipolar disorder. The world of parenting can be competitive and undermining. Probably most importantly, I had confidence in Joel as a parent, as well as a good support network of family, friends and work colleagues whose help I would seek out.

Around this time I recall receiving a letter inviting me to do jury service unless I was being treated for mental health issues. I responded to say that I was, and I received a second letter thanking me and telling me that they would never ask again. It seemed to be an extraordinarily discriminatory exclusion from the duties of a citizen. I understand, however, that the law on this has been rectified by the Mental Health (Discrimination) Act 2013. The Act took some years to pass because some politicians believed that it was not worth making amendments that would only affect two per cent of the people called up for jury service. That seems like a significant group of people to me.

When I am asked to fill in a questionnaire that asks if I have a disability, I have usually put no, as I am never sure if bipolar disorder counts as something as severe as physical or learning disabilities that permanently impact people. I am also never sure what the information will be used for and who might see it. Making choices about who to tell is quite different from having a label that, on its own, can have frightening and negative connotations for many people. History has not been kind to the mentally ill. I probably should answer yes to having a disability, as bipolar needs to be recognized, resourced and not hidden away. Solidarity with other disabled people who have fought hard and keep fighting for recognition and rights is something I have not done enough of on a personal level.

11
GIVING UP ON PSYCHIATRISTS

We moved again with a three-month interval at my Dad's cottage, which he was excited about, but I think we wore him out. A big attraction for the boys was always Grandad's sweets cupboard that he kept stocked with Kit Kats and Blue Ribands from the Nestle staff shop. This time the move was to a lovely 1920s house in Caterham with a wide, flat back garden that became very well-used. The elderly couple next door would confiscate footballs that went over, and we would apologize but just get new ones. Every month I went next door for tea by invitation, and I would take Oliver with his Woody doll from *Toy Story*. He remembers those teas as the most boring thing in his life. My neighbour would put on a 1950s frock and bake little cakes dispensed with doilies. It was really important to her.

Joel had a big pond dug into the garden that he filled with free koi carp from people who were moving and wanted to get rid of them. One day he looked out of the window and was alarmed to see a friend of Ben's, who had a few issues, trying to harpoon the fish with a bamboo cane. Generally, though, I think the fish led a contented life. Our neighbours took to coming through a gap in the hedge and sitting by the pond to look at the fish, which felt odd. On the other side was a really nice woman and her son, who later became a close friend of Ben's, but was so shy for the first year that we called him Boo Radley amongst ourselves. Our neighbours didn't get on, even before the single mum took in a heavily tattooed lodger who I was always defending. He was really nice.

Ben started primary school at the same one where my mother had taught before retiring and three of his cousins had attended. It was a five-minute walk away from the house and surrounded by a field. The area was semi-rural and green. It was nice to make friends with other parents on the playground, as it was a small, supportive school community linked to the church. We often had children back to play and held birthday parties for the whole class.

Oliver initially went to a nursery near the school, which we chose because it was warm and old-fashioned. Ben had been to a Montessori nursery that he really disliked, so we specifically looked for something different and less seemingly professional. Often when I picked him up, the staff would apologize deeply because the other children would have pulled his glasses flat, but it never seemed to bother Oliver. He made some lifelong friends there who went on to school with him.

My medical maintenance meant another GP and yet another psychiatrist. This time, the offices were on the grounds of a small hospital and looked as though they had been purpose-built more than 40 years previously, then abandoned. There was a reception area with a receptionist behind a screen. She was tiny but ruled the entrance with a rod of iron. She featured in a photograph on the wall – along with a much younger version of the psychiatrist – showing the opening of the centre. There were some petrified houseplants that looked as if they needed to be put out of their misery, and they may have featured in the photograph as well. Psychiatry is often referred to as the Cinderella of the health service, and that does tend to be reflected in the resources. The drugs prescribed were mostly developed in the 1950s and are ones that were developed to treat other conditions, then found to have a serendipitous effect, so nobody really knows how they work. Computers are often scarce or out of date, and prescriptions handwritten. Furniture is threadbare and carpets are coffee-stained. When people are feeling low, this type of environment doesn't help, and it does not convey confidence in the services. Staff do their best, but they, too, are in a low-priority service with low morale and a client group that is not always uplifting.

The psychiatrist was a nice man. With professionals, I knew he had a reputation for being difficult, but I found him courteous and reliable. I wanted to discuss changing from lithium to an alternative mood stabilizer, as a blood test had shown related thyroid issues. He tried hard to persuade me to continue lithium, as it was the Rolls Royce of mood stabilizers – I had often heard that said – and I could take medication for my thyroid. Then, he unexpectedly reeled off all the prescriptions he was taking for his complaints. It was as though something had finally snapped. Sadly, that was the last time I saw him, as he retired on health grounds, and the receptionist disappeared as well. The service they had proudly built up over years descended into chaos with a stream of locums. I stopped lithium and tried carbamazepine, which gave me a horrendous rash. I then tried lamotrigine, which was also a drug for epilepsy, and that seemed better. It was prescribed to me for seven days by a troubled-looking young psychiatrist in a leather jacket, and I was due to see him again on the seventh day. While he was asking me questions about sleep, I replied that I was suffering from brain chatter. This was an unwise comment that he interpreted not as a jokey remark but probably as confirmation of mental unwellness. On the seventh day a work commitment came up, and I phoned to ask if I could rearrange the appointment and pick up another prescription. The answer that came back was no. I went at the original appointment time to be told off like a naughty child for breaking an agreement that I had apparently made. He was angry and contemptuous. Always conscious of the power imbalance in the psychiatrist-patient relationship, I cooperated, but inside I was seething. I had to return again in two weeks, but this time, I kept my work social work ID badge on, and his whole attitude and demeanour was different. I told my GP that I no longer wanted to attend the resource centre, and he acknowledged that the service was having problems. I told him about my ID badge, and he laughed, but I pointed out that a lot of people aren't able to protect themselves in this way, and I have never had to since. My GP surgery has managed my situation since then, apart from a psychiatric consultation I requested about ten years later because I wanted to ask why I could not seem to manage without a large dose of sertraline alongside lamotrigine. My GP said the new psychiatrist was very good, but I was disappointed. He was late and wearing beads with jeans, which is no good for me, and it was in the usual sweaty, scruffy environment. My questions were put aside in favour of him taking a long history that was later reproduced in a letter with a major inaccuracy and a chunk missing. Quite some time later my issue was addressed by the GP surgery.

I have seen many psychiatrists over the years, and they have all been completely different. I don't know much about their training, but I don't think it can be very standardized or client-centred, as it seems to only occasionally produce a practitioner who naturally incorporates that approach as Dr O'Kane did. I find seeing a psychiatrist can be quite scary when I am ill because I feel vulnerable, and little is usually done to put me at ease, which could be down to time constraints. A dress code would help me to feel more respected – smart casual, fine.

Dad was a grandfather of 14 grandchildren with a wide age range. The two eldest cousins were Ben's godparents. My dad loved babies and would carry them around for hours, but as soon as they reached the age of two, he had high expectations of their independence. Dad continued to live in his cottage and served mass every morning. He was befriended by a strange and awkward priest who gave him a banana tree as a present. It was enormous and really belonged on a market stall, but Dad kept it in his small kitchen with two small bananas on it most of the time. Still a handsome man in his 80s, he was headhunted by a religious vestment company to model for their catalogue and paid with a cotter. He was often invited to lunches as the plus-one for the priest, who was sorely lacking in social skills. Dad was well-liked in the village and great company, but he always thought people were just being kind. He would attend ecumenical discussion groups with other churches and told me that Methodists were really nice with such a tone of surprise. I thought it a pity that Catholic segregation had been so dominant in his long life; he laughed about it. One summer we took him to France with us. At Dover there were a lot of small boats, but it was only when the ferry set sail that they announced it was the 50th anniversary of D-Day, and if there were any veterans on board, they could come up and accept a present. Dad said he didn't have any identification, but Joel ushered him up to meet the French captain who gave him a beautiful presentation box of Calvados. While we were in Normandy, we visited the beaches and saw the mulberry harbour that left him feeling introspective. He was able to find a church in which he had sheltered all those years ago. Dad didn't talk much about D-Day, but he said he was glad not to have been picked for the burial party.

As the years went by, we all met up for weddings, christenings and other events as a large family network, including camping in the New Forest for Dad's 80th birthday with a memorable game of rounders. Joel had borrowed a tent from his brother that turned out to be the size of Billy Smart's circus. My cousin Tim took it on as a challenge and organized everyone to put it up as the first of the day's activities. I think we just slept in the outer vestibule. Dad remained fit and strong into his 80s. He went to stay at Clare's for a few days, and she put absolutely all of his clothes in the washing machine. Initially cross, he then put on some of David's joggers and a sweatshirt, never to return to his old style. Sadly, Dad was diagnosed with bowel cancer and, although he was successfully operated on, he became ill again after two years. When I went to collect him from his cottage, he shed silent tears in the car, something I think he had learnt to do as a child. His ambition had always been to own his house, and now he was leaving it with Mum's toiletries still on her dressing table. He had to go into hospital with secondary lung cancer, and it was a job to get him out again. The doctor kept saying he needed scans and tests, but it was obvious he was dying, so we asked if that could be at home with us. Dad thought perhaps he was being experimented on. There was a story in the paper about a man who had both legs in plaster and was so desperate that his friends smuggled him out of hospital in the back of a van and took him to the pub. We considered kidnapping, but Dad was discharged suddenly, close to Christmas.

His old friends visited with their rosary beads to keep him company, and he would nod with the rosary when he could no longer talk. The priest dropped by often as the end was coming. One day I asked him if he could give Dad the last rites, and he had already done so at least five times. I had not understood that it was a prayer with an anointing to comfort the sick that had no purpose once death had taken place. Ben was eight, and Oliver was four years old. Dad liked watching them playing in the garden, as his bedroom was in the conservatory. Family members, including my nephew James, came and sat up with Dad through the night on a rota basis so that we could get some sleep. We knew when he was dying, as the GP had advised that his breathing would change. Clare arrived just in time to say goodbye, and he was gone. Three priests officiated Dad's funeral, which was an honour, and all the neighbours came. They decorated the church hall and put primulas on the tables, as these were the plants Dad always put on Mum's grave. The following day I took some flowers round to the agency who had provided his personal care, and the manager took me through to their office to see where someone had written on the whiteboard. It said, "RIP John Sheehan. A very nice man."

12
HEART SURGERY

Losing Dad was a huge blow, and I found myself exhausted from
caring for him while trying to prioritize the children. The GP
suggested sleeping tablets, but I declined and returned to work after
a couple of weeks. Work has always helped me in terms of structure,
and I get distracted by other people's issues. The important thing is
keeping them separate from your own.

A couple of years later, I began to experience mini strokes and saw
a cardiologist at East Surrey Hospital. He seemed unsure whether I
needed an MRI scan but decided that, as I had lost my speech on one
occasion, I should have one. When I received no result, I assumed
everything must be fine – until I had another mini stroke. This time
I was referred to Mayday Hospital, where a determined practitioner
wanted to get to the bottom of it. She obtained the MRI scan from
East Surrey, and it showed brain damage. It seemed the cardiologist
had walked out of his job due to pressures and funding issues while
my scan was filed. When I heard about the brain damage, I burst into
uncontrollable tears in the doctor's office. It was an uncharacteristic
response for me, and I think I was in shock. Taking lamotrigine
instead of lithium had never felt quite as stable, but I imagine that this
was a reaction anyone might have had. After various tests I was sent
for a last-ditch exploration in the form of a bubble test. The original
plan was for me to go with Joel, but a teacher training day crept up on
us and our neighbour, so we had three boys to take to Guy's Hospital
and a day out in London. I declined a sedative, as I didn't want to
be drowsy for the day, but I could see why it was offered. A spray

relaxed my muscles, and then an enormous pipe the size of a washing machine hose was put down my throat. Staying relaxed was a major feat. After a few minutes they found what they were looking for as bubbles of air passed through a hole in my heart, which I learnt had been there since birth. When I came out my partner said, "Nothing, then?" He had a healthy scepticism about my health issues, but I said I would have to have the hole closed.

I have always been much more worried about my mental health and taken my physical health for granted, but I think this was more relatable for him. That said, immediately in the wake of the September 11th attacks, he booked bargain flights for us all to go to Boston and ski in the White Mountains. The events of 9/11 were truly shocking, almost made for television. When I noticed Oliver flying his lego aeroplanes into buildings, we stopped watching the news. The boys took to skiing well, although their instructor asked me afterwards if they didn't talk to him because they thought he was a big, horrible American, a common fear Americans had as the world seemed set against them. I explained that they were just English and shy. We didn't see much of Joel on the slopes, as he was usually spotted boarding a snowmobile back to the lodge. We explored Boston and went to Salem. It was quite an adventure and the only time I have had my heels inspected before boarding a plane.

After a six-month wait, I had an operation at St George's Hospital to insert a tiny titanium umbrella into my heart that opened out to close the hole. The medics were really pleased with the outcome and suggested that I walk back to the ward afterwards. When I was taken down to the operating theatre, a young man pushed my wheelchair. He whizzed me around at great speed, and I wondered if he was doing community service. Walking back seemed a better plan after that, although the nursing staff were quite cross and felt the medics were showing off. The operation did make an immediate difference. I could breathe better, climb stairs more easily and had better colour, things that I had not realized were getting problematic. Plus, I had no more mini strokes or migraines. However, by this time, I could only conclude that I was born at the shallow end of the gene pool.

Returning to work was very strange. As soon as I logged onto my computer, a stark message came up that said I had been absent for over 12 days, so I had to see my service manager. I was shocked, and a friend who took me out for some air said ironically that it was enough to give someone a heart attack. I spoke to my service manager about receiving such a cold welcome back in an open-plan office, but he couldn't see the problem at all. That may have become standard practice in many businesses, but it was a cultural shift I didn't care for.

13
ANOTHER HOUSE MOVE

It was 2004 and time for another house move. Our public service salaries had stagnated – although we hadn't yet reached austerity – so moving up was one way to invest that had seemed to work so far. I think we also liked having a project. We made our way to a part of Caterham that we didn't know existed to see a house that we couldn't find in the woods. When we managed to link up with the estate agent, it was pouring with rain. The bungalow was a boxy 1950s corridor with little rooms, but the boys and their friends immediately went running off into the big woodland garden. That sold it to us. We had a creative financial adviser who enabled us to over-borrow, which was easily done at the time, and our existing house sold straight away to an architect. I loved that pretty house and took some comfort that it would be looked after, but when I was passing one day, they invited me in. Walls and doors had been moved, floorboards were covered with something synthetic and, even worse, the conservatory was bricked up. They wanted me to see what they had done, and I really had to dig deep for words of encouragement. Sometimes it's best not to go back.

We moved on a stormy February day, and Clare came to help. The previous owners were leaving to live near relatives, but they found it very hard to go and couldn't part with the keys. Joel sat with them at the estate agent's as it got later and later. The removal people had not actually seen the property, and their van barely made it up the steep hill before they encountered 50 feet of steps. By 9pm everything was in, including the piano, and most of it had stayed dry. The first night was amazing because there were no street lights, so it was pitch black with the sound of owls calling. I am so used to them now, I don't hear them unless I make a conscious effort. Ben had a friend round the next day – in fact, the harpoonist. That evening there was a knock on the door, and his mother, looking pale, disorientated and dishevelled, said she had to feel her way up the steps because there were no lights. It seemed very rural and perfect for the boys to play with their lightsabers. The garden was pretty overgrown, and I invited friends from work for a gardening party: all they could eat for all they could dig. There were loads of little statues of animals in the garden that the previous owners had left behind. I kept giving them to Joel's parents until his brother put his foot down over a large red fox.

We were only two miles from our previous home, but it seemed a world away, except that we didn't have to change schools, GP, football teams and so on. We met the people who built our house in 1955, and they explained that it was extended in stages when they could afford it, hence the utilitarian design. Neighbours were having changes to their homes that were all built on the hill in the 1930s and recommended an architect who suggested changes that really opened up our house. Our same financial adviser, quite a character, was able to stretch our mortgage to infinity, and we employed a motley crew of workers with their project manager to reconfigure the property. It was before online shopping, and we spent endless tortuous weekends on the Purley Way looking at kitchens and bathrooms. The kids hated it. Only one room remained untouched, so we spent six months basically camping in our own home. The saving grace was the banter that always made me laugh, but there were also endless feuds among the workers. Everyone hated the plumber and called him Leaky Pete. There was a really talented young plasterer who had learnt his trade in Ireland as a child, but he drank and would disappear. We kept asking if we could wait until he reappeared because his work was so good, but when he finally disappeared to Ireland to see a woman, he was sacked. Another young man without a specific role was impossibly clumsy but was the son of one of the company directors. When he broke the whisk, they made him mix the cement by hand,

and his days were numbered. Whatever the dramas and sackings of the day, they would all end up in the Golden Lion drinking together after work. It was a long six months with dust and dirt everywhere. The darkest time was when the bath was in the kitchen surrounded by holey dust sheets, and the kitchen sink was in the garden. A neighbour named Zoe came by and was shocked. She invited us all for a meal and has been a firm friend ever since. The renovation was worth it because the house is great, but it's not something I would readily do again with children.

14

ANOTHER CHALLENGE: MENOPAUSE

Things were becoming stressful at work. The building we had
really liked was being sold, and we were due to move to the central
office in Croydon. Hot-desking was a new concept that we strongly
objected to, and we said we would only move if we each had our
own desk. After many battles, we moved, and we each had a desk
with our name on it, but they were tiny. Impossibly, we were meant
to share one computer between two. The tightly packed rows of
desks filled an enormous factory-style space that had no dividers.
It was unrelenting and very noisy. Teams were mixed together. We
wondered if we were being punished for something, but I think
new styles of office management and cost-cutting were happening
everywhere. Managers came and went, while shrinking resources
put pressure on everyone – a familiar story in local authorities.

Some of my colleagues had left to work for a small voluntary
agency, and I applied to a different authority with better training and
resources. It was a steep learning curve, as their practice was much
better, and it was definitely the right move despite having to do a
lot of travelling. I worried about making the change to Surrey and
having a new medical declaration to make, but it was straightforward.
I really enjoyed the job and the people who were very innovative, but
decided after two years to take a job at the small voluntary agency
my former colleagues went to, as it was closer to home. It was not a
good move, and the giant crucifix should have given me a clue. It had
been a Catholic agency until the Equalities Act came into force and
meant they had to forego Catholic funding to recruit gay adopters.

The changes had not gone far enough. Gay adoption has been a great success story. Two years on I returned to Surrey with great relief despite the travelling, and I stayed until I retired. It was hard work but very satisfying.

During this time, life outside work continued to revolve around the boys. We went on holidays to Disney World and the Kennedy Space Center, which unfortunately ended Joel's willingness to fly. He was trapped next to a trolley in the aisle for an hour on a cramped Virgin flight during turbulence, and he developed claustrophobia. We did fly once more to Gran Canaria, but he had to take copious amounts of Valium that he didn't like to get home again. Thereafter, we had driving holidays to France and Spain with *Harry Potter* CDs to keep us all going. Those were some of my favourite trips because we really got to see the countries. Ben and Oliver learnt to swim well, and Oliver played the piano reluctantly. Joel's parents came to a concert that Oliver was playing in, but we had to wrestle away a bag of Hula Hoops from his mum, who was crunching loudly and saying she was bored. In fact, she was becoming unwell and died soon afterwards from a blocked heart valve that had stopped her from breathing properly and caused some effects similar to Alzheimer's. Joel's dad, a very gentle and personable man, died some years later, and it was a big loss for the boys. The parents had come to us for every Christmas and Easter, and Joel's brothers still come. When he came for his last Christmas, Joel's dad was in a wheelchair, and when everyone was carrying him out to the car, they became wedged between walls and couldn't move because they were laughing so hard. Ben and Oliver were shocked to hear their gentle Grandad swearing. The wakes for Joel's parents were held at our house and gave us rare chances to see extended family and catch up.

Oliver loved football and played with local teams. I spent most weekends driving him to matches all over Surrey. He bought me a folding chair and Thermos mug for my birthday, thus ensuring that I would keep going despite some very vocal, badly behaved parents trying to relive their glory days through their children. On one occasion, a young manager argued endlessly with the referee until he was ordered to go and stand under a distant tree. Two other parents were sent there as well, and it was very funny, but made a serious point. Both boys went on to a secondary school that, unusually, was Catholic, Church of England and Free Faith. The thing that I valued the most was that they both had very good friends and still do.

The menopause was a struggle for me as it had been for my mum. It seemed to kickstart when I had heart surgery. Like periods and sanitary products, it felt like a strange, hidden rite of passage. Aside from throwing cardigans off and on, I would lose track of what I was about to say when I became aware that a hot flush was coming. This was disastrous in a meeting, when giving evidence at court or on any other number of occasions. On top of managing bipolar fluctuations in mood that still happened despite medication, the menopause was challenging. I was not a candidate for Hormone Replacement Therapy, but if I had been, I would have taken it. The GP told me that my symptoms could last up to a year, and a friend at work just looked at me knowingly. Ten years later, it has calmed down, but I don't think my thermostat has ever been the same. The onset started in the dreaded open-plan office in Croydon, where the sun would beat down on the flat roof, and the windows were locked shut with no blinds. During a heatwave when the temperature soared, I tackled the manager, and he told me jokingly to talk to the director, which I did. She came down and demanded air-conditioning units and that I was kept informed of progress. It felt like a glimpse of female solidarity. The manager muttered that 20 air-conditioning units were now coming out of his budget, but it was a little triumph that suited the largely female staff group.

It was hard to sleep during the menopause, and the general level of exhaustion was difficult. On top of that were the occasional periods of depression. A feeling of gloomy detachment, hollow sadness and ineptitude might be the first signs, along with a sense that the world was black and white instead of colour. I would always let some friends or colleagues know when I was struggling, but I would plough on as best I could, relieved by drug therapy for months. Knowing who to tell about my bipolar and get a positive reaction tended to be instinctive, although I didn't really mind anyone knowing at this stage in my life. When I returned to Surrey, I was due to provide some training to a large group with a newly qualified colleague who I didn't know well. I'd had a change in medication and thought I better tell her, as I didn't know if it had taken effect. I did know that she was warm and inclusive. The group was about to start, and Gina opened her eyes wide and said, "Timing, Brigid. Timing." The four days went really well. I think I might have been a bit manic, but that can work well with a crowd. Gina was great.

Then, an additional problem came with frequent bouts of cystitis that were quite debilitating for several years. Lots of investigations showed that it was not caused by infection, but it was more of a bladder irritation. It seemed a mystery to various GPs who assumed it was somehow menopause-related, but an excellent nurse practitioner worked through all the medications I was taking and concluded that the cause was lamotrigine. I had also started to wonder how effective it still was as a mood stabilizer because I seemed to be taking greater amounts of the antidepressant sertraline without being able to reduce it. One GP suggested that I was suffering from anxiety more than depression, as it was primarily a drug for anxiety. Another suggested trying an anti-epileptic drug called pregabalin instead of lamotrigine, as there seemed to be a reluctance to prescribe lithium, which is hard on the system. Pregabalin has a euphoric effect, and I found myself feeling completely stoned. While off work, I must admit I enjoyed the sensation of not caring about anything at all, but I couldn't carry on in that state. My manager from Surrey came to see me, and I could tell she felt surprised. I went through a process with occupational health, who were very helpful and put a managed return to work in place. The practitioner who I saw was specifically qualified in mental health, and my apprehension turned to relief as we were both on the same page.

With my GP I became insistent on going back to lithium and, after taking advice from a psychiatrist, he organized it with a blood test. I stopped getting cystitis and felt much better on lithium. It seems that there is no one psychiatric drug that can be consistently relied on throughout the lifespan, simply because the effects are cumulative, and other influences like pregnancy, age and menopause have an impact. I have read that the painkiller pregabalin is a class-C drug with a street value and is used by heroin addicts to enhance the effect. The world of psychiatric medicine often feels hit and miss to me. It is difficult to assert yourself to confidently challenge treatment offered, or to have faith in psychiatric services that seem rigidly hierarchical and have changed little for decades. Stigma and debilitating illness stop sufferers from demanding better, and few people seem motivated, willing or able to listen in the face of competing priorities.

15

RETIREMENT

A year ago I retired with impeccable timing as COVID-19 appeared. Two years ago there was a tragic death of a young person at work that I found really upsetting, and I started to feel very weary. I knew that I had reached the end, so I set a date to retire in a year with plenty of notice to colleagues, as well as time for me to make an adjustment and complete my work. I no longer felt I could do a good job. As I was born in the 50s, it was not ideal from a pension point of view, but we thought we would manage. Joel had already taken redundancy and spent the first three months asleep on the sofa. Social work takes its toll. We both planned to do some sessional work but couldn't face the stress once we had got used to not having it. My expectation had always been to retire at 60, then suddenly 62, and, finally, 66, but I couldn't keep going that long. I don't think men's pensions would be changed in such a cavalier fashion. I decided to have some work-based counselling for myself and found it much more useful than I had expected. It was a short course of sessions that looked at endings and responsibilities with a life map that I was asked to compile. I felt validated by it and as though I had choices.

I have followed the medical model in terms of medication throughout my adult life, and perhaps I have not been brave enough to risk family, job and home to try alternatives, apart from the one experience in Canada, which was certainly a deterrent. I tend to agree with current wisdom that suggests a combination of talking and drug therapy is probably beneficial for bipolar disorder. I could not have managed without drug therapy despite its side effects, but many do. Some people have told me that drugs rob them of their identity, and that the highs can be really enjoyable. Basically, it's whatever gets you through your life.

I had a lovely send-off from friends and colleagues who I miss, but the sense of freedom is fantastic. After starting school at age four and working until 64, time is no longer regimented. Waking up in the morning with no pressure and no casework rattling around in my head leaves me feeling as though the weight of the world has been lifted. I don't think I had realized how hard I had to work on so many levels just to keep up.

In March 2020 I went with my sons – but sadly without Joel, who just couldn't fly – to visit Clare at her home in Seattle with plans to go to Oregon, all to celebrate my retirement. However, COVID-19 was surfacing, and Clare was deeply worried about the virus. She kept reading us the terrifying news reports from Italy on social media. So, Oliver took charge and, just ahead of the curve, we caught the early morning train across the US border to Vancouver, and he booked us a terrific Airbnb above a tattoo parlour downtown. The train route was closed down the following day. We booked earlier flights back to the UK and then had three days to explore. Crisp, cold and sunny, Vancouver was just as beautiful as I remembered, and the boys loved it. We walked everywhere and had some great meals, including at Bridges Restaurant on Granville Island, which hadn't changed at all. I looked for the Women's Resources Centre on Robson Street and thought it had gone, but came across its new premises in Robson Square, which had been opened by Dr Ruth Sigal. We hoped to be able to go to the pub on St Patrick's Day, but the lockdown started and we flew out the next day. It wasn't what I had in mind, but I really enjoyed it while it lasted.

The flight via Calgary was quite tense because everyone was alarmed by the pandemic about which we knew so little. The cabin crew kept pouring us free drinks until the gin and tonic ran out. We arrived home safely to find that Joel had kitted out the house with every possible medical aid and masses of toilet roll. Lockdowns have come and gone since then, and we are just waiting patiently for whatever the future holds, punctuated by Zoom gatherings and WhatsApps that feed the soul.

In looking over the part that bipolar disorder has played in my life, I realize it has been considerable. It makes me sad to think what might have been possible without it.

Brigid Sheehan
April 2021

ACKNOWLEDGEMENTS

Elaine Skinner, a dear friend, who was the first person to read this book and to think it had possibilities. Elaine gave constructive advice and encouragement.

James Spackman, my nephew, for his sound, honest advice on publishing and content.

Thomas McGrath, designer and artist, for his cover ideas and technical help.

My son Oliver for his patience, if not understanding, with my laptop issues.

All my family and friends who have been with me through thick and thin, with a special mention for Julie, my oldest friend.

Cherish Editions and Trigger Publishing.

ABOUT CHERISH EDITIONS

Cherish Editions is a bespoke self-publishing service for authors of mental health, wellbeing and inspirational books.

As a division of Trigger Publishing, the UK's leading independent mental health and wellbeing publisher, we are experienced in creating and selling positive, responsible, important and inspirational books, which work to de-stigmatize the issues around mental health and improve the mental health and wellbeing of those who read our titles.

Founded by Adam Shaw, a mental health advocate, author and philanthropist, and leading psychologist Lauren Callaghan, Cherish Editions aims to publish books that provide advice, support and inspiration. We nurture our authors so that their stories can unfurl on the page, helping them to share their uplifting and moving stories.

Cherish Editions is unique in that a percentage of the profits from the sale of our books goes directly to leading mental health charity Shawmind, to deliver its vision to provide support for those experiencing mental ill health.

Find out more about Cherish Editions by visiting cherisheditions.com or by joining us on:

Twitter @cherisheditions
Facebook @cherisheditions
Instagram @cherisheditions

Cherish
EDITIONS

ABOUT SHAWMIND

A proportion of profits from the sale of all Trigger books go to their sister charity, Shawmind, also founded by Adam Shaw and Lauren Callaghan. The charity aims to ensure that everyone has access to mental health resources whenever they need them.

You can find out more about the work Shawmind do by visiting shawmind.org or joining them on:

Twitter @Shaw_Mind

Facebook @ShawmindUK

Instagram @Shaw_Mind

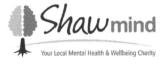

Your Local Mental Health & Wellbeing Charity

Lightning Source UK Ltd.
Milton Keynes UK
UKHW040629091221
395374UK00001B/4

9 781913 615505